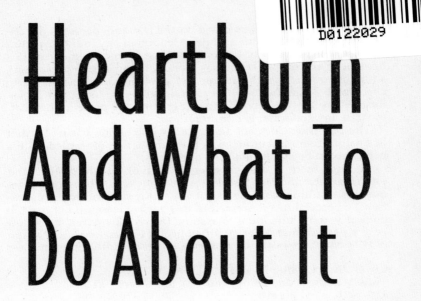

Heartburn And What To Do About It

Dr. James F. Balch
Dr. Morton Walker

A DR. MORTON WALKER HEALTH BOOK

AVERY
a member of Penguin Putnam Inc.

The advice in this book is based on the training, personal experiences, and research of the authors. Mention of any individual clinician should in no way be construed as an endorsement of this book or of any of the techniques therein. Because each person and situation are unique, the author and publisher urge the reader to check with a qualified health professional before using any procedure where there is any question regarding the presence or treatment of any abnormal health condition.

The publisher does not advocate the use of any particular diet or health program, but believes the information presented in this book should be available to the public.

Because there is always some risk involved, the author and publisher are not responsible for any adverse effects or consequences resulting from the use of any of the suggestions, preparations, or procedures described in this book. Please do not use the book if you are unwilling to assume the risk. Feel free to consult with a physician or other qualified health professional. It is a sign of wisdom, not cowardice, to seek a second or third opinion.

Cover design: Doug Brooks,
  Eric Macaluso, and Rudy Shur
Typesetters: Al Berotti
  and Elaine V. McCaw
In-house editor: Lisa James

Avery
a member of
Penguin Putnam Inc.
375 Hudson Street
New York, NY 10014
www.penguinputnam.com

Library of Congress Cataloging-in-Publication Data

Balch, James F., 1933–
   Heartburn and what to do about it : a guide to overcoming
the discomforts of indigestion using drug-free remedies / by
James F. Balch, Morton Walker.
      p. cm.
   Includes bibliographical references and index.
   ISBN 0-89529-792-2 (pbk.)
   1. Indigestion—Popular works.   2. Heartburn—Popular works.
I. Walker, Morton. II. Title.
RC827.B35 1998
616.3'32—dc21   97-46876
                                                        CIP

Printed in the United States of America

10   9   8   7   6   5   4

Contents

From Morton Walker, D.P.M.:
To Charlie Fox, a loving man,
who has done good deeds ever since I've known
him for these past twenty-eight years,
as well as long before we came together.
This is Charlie's Book!

From James Balch, M.D.:
I too have known the goodness and love of Charlie Fox.
Without his influence and caring,
this work would not have happened.
Thank you, Charlie.

Foreword

Heartburn is a tremendous problem in this country. Americans spend enormous sums of money each year to relieve heartburn symtomatically, be it with acid-blocking drugs or with antacids. But heartburn is not an acid-blocking drug deficiency. Many of these drugs interfere with nutrient absorption and give the body yet another synthetic chemical to detoxify. Worst of all, these drugs do not help in the long term: They do not solve the problem right at the source, and they often cause more problems than they solve. This leads to a lot of needless suffering—suffering that could have been alleviated if natural medicine had been used in the first place. The same can be said of other digestive complaints, ranging from nausea to constipation.

I was, therefore, very pleased when I heard that Drs. Balch and Walker were writing their new book, *Heartburn and What to Do About It*. One of the most important tenets of natural medicine is that of removing the offending cause which is at the root of an ailment. In this groundbreaking book, the authors insist that you solve the problem of heartburn by getting to the root cause. You can read about the many possible causes that can lie behind this painful and annoying problem, and behind other common digestive problems, in this comprehensive guide.

You will also learn a very important lesson: how your digestive tract works. Once you see how these important organs function so well and in such harmony when you eat the right diet, take the right supplements, have the right bacterial population in your digestive tract, and manage stress, you will understand the power of natural medicine and healthy living. Your body wants to be healthy, and that includes your digestive tract. Once you support its function in the manner that Drs. Balch and Walker recommend, you will have the healthy and smooth-running digestive system you desire.

Every case of heartburn is different, and the same is true of other digestive problems. That is why I am so excited that this book covers all the territory you need to examine in order to root out the many possible causes of illness. There is an excellent discussion of the importance of having the right bacteria, the friendly bacteria your body needs, in the digestive tract. This is paramount! As a nutritionist, time and again I have seen the presence of proper intestinal bacteria play a key role in enhancing bowel health and eliminating heartburn.

I am also pleased that there is an in-depth discussion of parasites, a possible root cause of disease that many people neglect when trying to alleviate their digestive problems. Parasites may seem like an unpleasant topic, but it is far more unpleasant to let such a problem go untreated. I have seen many cases of chronic heartburn clear up only when an antiparasite strategy was adopted. The same can be said of chronic yeast overgrowth, another topic explored in this book. The presence of either excessive *Candida albicans* or parasites must be addressed if heartburn and other ailments are to be truly eliminated.

The bigger picture presented by this book is the importance of optimal digestion. If you follow the suggestions outlined by the authors, you will do more than just eliminate heartburn and other disorders. You will maximize the health of your digestive tract, and in so doing promote the health of your entire body in myriad ways. Only when we are properly breaking down, absorbing, and assimilating food can we enjoy the highest level of health.

If you have heartburn, buy this book. Buy another one for your doctor. Discuss the many strategies that you can use to attack this and other digestive problems by getting to their root causes. When you do, your body will be much healthier and happier, and you will experience the victory over illness that only natural healing can deliver.

Robert Crayhon, M.S.
Author of The Carnitine Miracle
New Rochelle, New York

Introduction

Are you living with chronic heartburn? You may not know it, but your problems may result from a war being waged within your digestive tract, a war between friendly, health-enhancing bacteria and hostile, disease-causing bacteria. To remain in good shape, your gastrointestinal system must remain in balance, with the helpful microbes keeping the harmful invaders in check. If this balance is upset, you may suffer from such common digestive complaints as heartburn, with its associated gas and bloating, or from other problems, such as constipation or diarrhea. These discomforts, bad enough in and of themselves, may indicate the presence of more serious conditions, such as ulcers, several inflammatory bowel diseases, irritable bowel syndrome, or even various parasitic infections.

Unfortunately, life in the modern fast lane both creates and aggravates indigestion. It creates problems because many of us habitually consume junk food, such as hot dogs, potato chips, and pastries, instead of nourishing food, such as fresh vegetables and fruits, whole grains, and yogurt. A poor diet can reduce levels of beneficial bacteria within the intestines, so that the disease-causing bacteria tend to take over. This problem is amplified by the stressful lifestyle many of us endure, and by disease, injury, and pollution.

Modern life then aggravates digestive troubles by offering short-term solutions, such as antacids and other nonprescription medications. These remedies may offer immediate relief, but, over time, are likely to create more problems than they solve by causing a rebound effect, in which the original symptoms reappear, or by masking the signs of serious digestive-system damage.

A hectic lifestyle and over-the-counter drugs are not the only causes of indigestion. People of middle age or older often have diminished levels of hydrochloric acid, a condition known as hypochlorhydria, or a complete lack of acid, known as achlorhydria. These people have a hard time digesting meat protein. According to the United States Department of Agriculture, about 40 percent of American women over the age of fifty have hypochlorhydria, which leaves them susceptible to infections such as stomach flu.[1]

In addition, antibiotics and other medicines upset the balance of bacteria within the gastrointestinal tract. Of course, you know that the nature of antibiotics is to kill harmful bacteria, but—and this is a big disadvantage connected with antibiotics—though they have worked wonders against many diseases, antibiotics also kill helpful good bacteria at the same time. These good bacteria help the body both to digest food and to defend itself against disease. Eliminating the good microbes leads to pathological conditions such as the yeast syndrome.[2]

In the first part of this book, we will examine the scope of the indigestion problem before discussing specific digestive problems, including separate chapters on ulcers (Chapter 4), bacterial imbalance (Chapter 5), the leaky gut syndrome (Chapter 6), the yeast syndrome (Chapter 7), and intestinal parasites (Chapter 8). In the second part, we will offer natural, safe solutions to the indigestion problem, including proper diet (Chapter 9, with a separate discussion of yogurt in Chapter 10) and internal cleansers (Chapter 11).

Finally, in Chapter 12, we will turn to the topic of supplementation with friendly—or *probiotic*—bacteria. We will tell you what species are most helpful, what they do, what to look for in a supplement, and how supplements should be taken. We believe that supplementation with probiotics is an absolute requirement for good intestinal health. It is also a vital part of overall health, since, as we will see, probiotic bacteria serve functions that go far beyond the digestive tract.

You need never suffer from indigestion again. We invite you to learn how in the following pages.

PART ONE

Indigestion Problems

Indigestion strikes almost everyone at some time or another—after a particularly large meal, let us say, or during an unusually busy week. But if your usual glass of the sparkling bubbly is two fizzy tablets in water, you are probably one of the millions of people who suffer from chronic indigestion, with its pain, heartburn, and bloating. There is a wide range of possible reasons for abdominal discomfort. Some are minor, some are not. It is important to know the difference.

In this part, we will discuss the size of the indigestion problem, and provide an overview of the disorders that affect the digestive tract. We will then describe some of the more troublesome disorders—including ulcers, a state of imbalance called dysbiosis, the leaky gut and yeast syndromes, and intestinal parasites—with an emphasis on natural methods of treatment. So stop reaching for those antacids, and start learning what may really be ailing you.

CHAPTER 1

The Size of the Indigestion Problem

Do you suffer from heartburn and bloating, abdominal cramps and gas, or other forms of indigestion? If you do, you are not alone. Each year, about 12 million Americans are prompted to visit their doctors with digestive complaints. Many experience digestive problems so regularly that they use over-the-counter medications on an ongoing basis. Some are found to be suffering from diseases, such as irritable bowel syndrome or ulcers, that require medical attention (see "When to Call the Doctor" on page 8). There is no doubt about it—indigestion is a serious problem.

In this chapter, we will first look at what lifestyle factors are linked to digestive problems, and at the hard-fought marketplace battle for digestive-aid dollars. We will then see why over-the-counter medications do not work.

LIFESTYLE AND THE INCIDENCE OF DIGESTIVE PROBLEMS

Recently, a survey was done by the Simmons Market Research Bureau (SMRB) on who tends to buy the most di-

When to Call the Doctor

Most abdominal troubles are not serious and respond well to self-care. But if you are also experiencing weight loss, chronic fever, or any of the following symptoms and signs, you should call your doctor:

- *Sudden, persistent change in bowel habits.* This might indicate inflammatory bowel disease, or colon or possibly pancreatic cancer.

- *Constipation that comes on suddenly and persists.* This might indicate diverticulosis, irritable bowel syndrome, or colon cancer, particularly if the stools are bloody.

- *Vomiting.* This might indicate food poisoning; gallbladder disease; ulcers; intestinal obstruction, if defecation is impossible; appendicitis, if the pain is in the lower-right abdomen; or stomach cancer, if the vomit is bloody or there is constant pain in the upper abdomen.

- *Chronic and severe abdominal pain.* This might indicate irritable bowel syndrome; peptic ulcer; stomach cancer; pancreatitis or pancreatic cancer, if the pain is in the upper abdomen; gallbladder disease, if the pain is in the upper-right abdomen; diverticulosis; ulcerative colitis; Crohn's disease; colon cancer, if the pain is in the lower abdomen; intestinal obstruction; appendicitis; aneurysm; peritonitis; food poisoning; or hernia.

- *Abdominal swelling.* This might indicate intestinal obstruction, if there is also severe pain is in the lower abdomen.

- *Loss of bowel control.* This may indicate acute diarrhea, food poisoning, fecal impaction, or colon cancer.

- *Heartburn unrelieved by antacids.* This may indicate hiatus hernia, ulcers, gallbladder disease, or cancer of the esophagus or stomach, or possibly a heart attack.

- *Bloody or black stools.* This may indicate hemorrhoids, anal fissures, ulcers, diverticular disease, ulcerative colitis, or stomach or colon cancer.

- *Pale stools.* This may indicate a gallbladder or liver disorder.

- *Inability to defecate.* This may indicate an intestinal obstruction.

Source: S. Rees. Stomachaches: when to worry, what to do. *Family Circle*, 14 March 1995, p. 39.

---

gestive aids, and where they tend to live.[1] When combined with information gathered jointly by the market survey firm A.C. Nielsen and the drug company SmithKline Beecham, one of the leading manufacturers of nonprescription digestive aids, the survey provides a rather detailed profile of the typical American indigestion sufferer.

One conclusion the SMRB reached is that most people who have heartburn live in the South, with Virginia topping the list. (Second place went to West Virginia.) According to the survey results, the incidence of heartburn—technically known as *stomach acid reflux*—is at least 20 percent higher in the southeastern United States than anywhere else in the country.

The SMRB survey revealed other interesting facts. For example, women suffer more indigestion than men, and older people more than younger people. Residents of rural areas tend to buy more digestive aids than residents of urban or suburban areas. On the other hand, urbanites tend to suffer more problems with gas than suburbanites. People in the middle-income brackets—from $30,000 to $60,000 a year—tend to have more indigestion than people in the upper or lower income ranges. The same thing goes for full-time workers versus part-time workers. Skilled blue collar workers and clerical or sales workers have less indigestion than managers and other professionals. Better-educated people tend to have more indigestion than lesser-educated people. Homeowners are worse off than renters. Finally, people who live with children also tend to buy more digestive aids than those who have no children in the household.

THE BATTLE FOR THE AMERICAN INDIGESTION DOLLAR

One only has to watch a night's worth of television to see the battle being fought by the giant pharmaceutical firms, and their advertising agencies, for the digestive-aid market in the United States. There is a good reason: A lot of money is at stake. Over-the-counter stomach soothers rank just behind painkillers and on a par with cold remedies in the space they occupy on the nation's medicine shelf. In 1995, Americans spent $1.7 billion on antacids, and their total purchases tripled in 1996 as a result of heartburn products called histamine-II (H2) blockers. These include drugs such as famotindine (Pepcid AC), ranitidine (Zantac 75), cimetidine (Tagamet HB), nizatidine (Axid), and omeprazole (Prilosec).

The H2-blocker battles began when Tagamet, a prescription ulcer drug, was nearing the end of its patent protection. Since loss of the patent would mean competition from low-priced generic copies, the drug's maker, SmithKline Beecham, developed a milder version of Tagamet, brand-named Tagamet HB—the *HB* stands for "heartburn"—that could be advertised and sold without a prescription. Two other manufacturers of popular ulcer treatments followed suit, and produced Pepcid AC and Zantac 75. Others, drawn by the lucrative market, eventually created and brought out their own H2-blocker products.

This started a race to meet with United States Food and Drug Administration (FDA) approval and get these new products into the stores. The scramble for shelf space was backed by millions of dollars in print and electronic media advertising. The various companies offered all sorts of promotions and discounts, and competed for endorsements, awards, and approvals from semigovernmental agencies. Health maintenance organizations, in an effort to cut costs, started advising their participating doctors to switch heartburn and gastric ulcer patients away from prescription drugs and into the cheaper, nonprescription versions.

Each manufacturer asserted that its product was vastly superior to any competitors. They all claimed faster, more complete relief of heartburn. Not surprisingly, the fight spilled into the courts, with companies accusing each other of false advertising.[2]

All of this money and effort might have been (and continue to be) well spent, if H2 blockers were the answer to the problem. They are not.

DIGESTIVE AIDS CAN ACTUALLY CAUSE DIGESTIVE DISTRESS

Acid indigestion results when the stomach's contents back up into the esophagus, stinging sensitive tissue. The muscle that lies between the stomach and esophagus usually closes to prevent such reflux. Sometimes, though, the muscle fails to close properly. There are a number of possible reasons, including overeating, stress, smoking, pregnancy, excess weight, and lying down before a meal has sufficiently digested. Certain foods can also cause heartburn. Fatty foods, alcohol, and chocolate can all temporarily weaken the gateway. Alcoholic beverages and spicy or acidic foods can irritate the digestive passages directly. Among the worst heartburn triggers are caffeinated drinks, because they stimulate the production of gastric acid.

Unlike antacids, which make the stomach's contents less acidic, H2 blockers actually reduce the body's production of stomach acid. (That is why antacids are taken after meals, while H2 blockers are taken before meals.) Unfortunately, it takes a while for H2 blockers to take effect. And a major concern is that they can mask the symptoms of either an active ulcer or—much worse—cancer of the stomach or esophagus.[3]

H2 blockers can also produce various side effects. For example, cimetidine can cause breast enlargement in men and mental confusion in older people, among other effects. Other H2 blockers have their own potential side effects. These effects are more likely to occur when prescription-strength dosages are taken, but may result in problems even at the lower dosages used in nonprescription drugs.

Antacid use is not the answer to the indigestion problem, either. Some manufacturers of antacids make a point of claiming "fast, fast, fast relief," but tests carried out by the staff of *Consumer Reports* found little difference in how rapidly the tested products go to work. When they bring comfort, it is because the contents of the stomach is elevated to a pH of 3.0 or higher.[4] The pH scale measures acidity: the lower the number, the more acidic the substance, with neutral being seven.

Antacids are made of several kinds of ingredients. One ingredient is simethicone. Simethicone is said to allow small gas bubbles in the digestive tract to coalesce into bigger ones, which are presumably easier to expel. However, a panel of outside experts convened by the FDA concluded that there is insufficient data to support the claim by manufacturers about the ingredient's effectiveness against gas.

Sodium bicarbonate, a common antacid ingredient, contains more than 1,100 milligrams of sodium, nearly half the recommended daily maximum for a healthy adult. This amount of sodium is an unhealthy excess for people who must watch their sodium intake, including those with high blood pressure or congestive heart failure.

Bicarbonate by itself can cause a disturbance in the chemical balance of the blood. Bicarbonate supports urinary tract infections by making the urine too alkaline. Also, some users can experience ruptured stomach when they take bicarbonate after a big meal. The FDA has already recorded several deaths from bicarbonate usage.

Some antacids are made with calcium. It is true that everyone needs calcium, especially postmenopausal women, and that antacids can provide from 20 to 40 percent of the 1,000 milligrams of calcium recommended daily for an adult. But that does not mean that you should take a *drug*, which contains a number of ingredients, to do the work of a *supplement*. Calcium-based antacids may cause *acid rebound*, in which the stomach produces even more heartburn-inducing gastric acid after the antacid has exhausted itself.

Magnesium hydroxide and magnesium carbonate are other ingredients used in antacids. Both have a laxative effect, so they are often combined with aluminum compounds, which tend to be constipating. Unfortunately, aluminum can accumulate in the brain and eventually lead to Alzheimer's disease, especially among older people who have experienced a decline in kidney function. The magnesium in these antacids can also affect people with kidney trouble. Damaged kidneys do not eliminate all the magnesium, so the mineral will accumulate to cause high blood pressure, as well as heartbeat and respiration problems.[5] Moreover, long-term use of aluminum-containing antacids can rob the body of calcium. This weakens bones, resulting in osteoporosis.

Antacids may interfere with the action of certain drugs. By lowering the amount of stomach acid, antacids cause some coated pills to release their active ingredient earlier than intended—in the stomach, rather than in the small intestine. Antacids also tend to accelerate or inhibit the absorption into the bloodstream of some prescription drugs. For instance, one should never take them with tetracycline or similar antibiotics. Other drugs that do not mix well with antacids include diuretics, anticonvulsants, tranquilizers, and iron supplements.

No wonder nutritional supplement expert Earl Mindell, R.Ph., Ph.D., says: "Manufacturers won't admit it—but their antacids are often the cause of chronic stomach pain. Please don't take antacids for indigestion. . . . You can beat indigestion naturally."[6]

As you can see, you should think twice before reaching for that bottle in the medicine cabinet. Digestive aids are often ineffective, or worse. In this book, we will describe better ways of easing digestive problems. First, though, let us take a closer look at the types of problems that afflict the digestive system.

CHAPTER 2

Problems in the Upper Digestive Tract

The digestive system is affected by a wide range of acute and chronic illnesses. Some of these illnesses are fairly common, such as ulcers and hepatitis. Others, such as cystic fibrosis, inflammatory bowel diseases, and pancreatitis, occur less frequently, but with effects that may be just as devastating. More Americans are hospitalized for digestive disorders than for any other type of illness. Digestive illness costs billions of dollars in direct health care costs and additional billions in lost work time and productivity.

When people think about serious medical problems in the upper gastrointestinal (GI) tract, they generally think of ulcers. However, ulcers are just one of the health problems that can plague this part of the digestive system. Every year, about 31 million Americans are chronically ill with diseases of the upper GI tract.

In this chapter, after a quick review of the organs and functions of the upper GI tract, we will look at the disorders that affect this part of the body, while in the next chapter, we will look at the disorders that affect the lower GI tract. (For more information on a specific disorder or organ, contact the appropriate organization in Appendix A.)

ANATOMY AND FUNCTION OF THE UPPER GI TRACT

The upper GI tract includes the mouth, esophagus, stomach, liver, pancreas, and duodenum (see Figure 2.1). Food enters the mouth, where it is reduced to small bits by chewing and where *saliva* starts to break down carbohydrates, thus beginning the process of digestion. Food then travels through the throat, down the esophagus, and through the *gastroesophageal constrictor*, the thickened muscle at the bottom of the esophagus, before entering the stomach. The stomach serves as a storage organ and as the place where acidic *gastric juices* begin to break down proteins. The stomach also secretes a substance that allows vitamin B_{12} (cobalamin) to be absorbed.

The stomach is divided into three parts. The top of the stomach, called the *fundus*, lies above the opening from the esophagus. The middle two-thirds of the stomach is called the *body*. The lower third is called the *pyloric antrum*.

Food then passes into the duodenum, which is actually about the first foot or so of the small intestine. At that point, it encounters *pancreatic juice*, which is secreted by the pancreas. This juice stops the action of the stomach acids and readies the food for the small intestine. The food is also met by *bile*, which is secreted by the liver and stored in the gallbladder. Bile helps break down fats.

The entire GI tract is lined by a *mucous membrane*. This membrane secretes some of the digestive fluids found in various parts of the tract. It also secretes mucus to moisten and protect the digestive tract. The mucous membrane lies on top of a layer called the *submucosa*, which nourishes and supports it. In the esophagus, stomach, and duodenum, the submucosa lies on top of a layer of muscle called the *muscularis externia*, which serves to propel food along the tract in a wave-like motion called *peristalsis*. The entire package is wrapped in a tough, fibrous layer called the *serosa*. The lower GI tract is also made up of these four layers.

DISORDERS AFFECTING THE UPPER GI TRACT

For the average person, *indigestion* is that unpleasant group of sensations and symptoms that arise from somewhere in the upper GI tract, and include upper abdominal discomfort or pain located just below the breastbone. In addition, common sensations include abdominal distention, fullness, and bloating, sometimes accompanied by belching, nausea, and even vomiting. Gastroenterologists, those doctors who specialize in diseases of the GI tract, use the term *dyspepsia* to refer to this collection of symptoms.

In this section, we will look at disorders that affect the upper GI tract.

Mouth, Throat, and Esophagus Disorders

These ailments include:

- *Disorders of the mouth,* including inflammation and dry mouth

- *Disorders of the esophagus,* including swallowing disorders and esophageal varices, or enlarged veins located in the esophagus

- *Heartburn (stomach acid reflux),* irritation and inflamma-

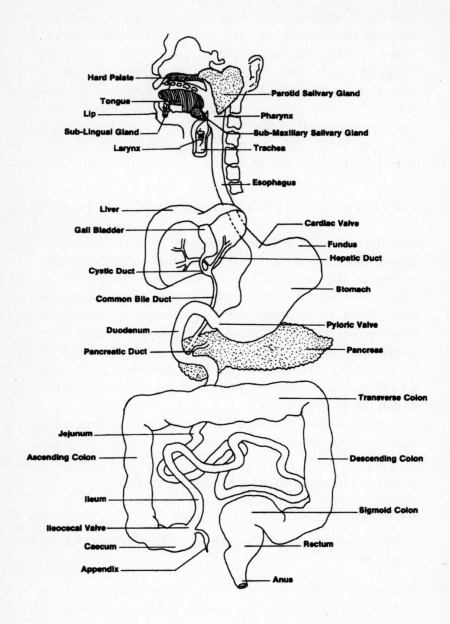

Figure 2.1. The Gastrointestinal Tract

tion due to the backwash of stomach contents into the esophagus

- *Hiatus hernia*, a condition in which part of the stomach slides up through the diaphragm into the chest cavity

There are several conditions, beside various dental problems, that can affect the mouth. The mucous membranes of the mouth may become inflamed, resulting in a condition called *stomatitis*. This can happen as the result of recurrent mouth ulcers; thrush, an oral form of candida infection (see Chapter 7); bacterial or viral infections; tumors, either benign or malignant; or poorly fitting dentures. Dry mouth, also known as *xerostomia*, may be caused by persistent mouth-breathing, dehydration, or certain kinds of drugs. Offensive breath may result from poor dental hygiene, smoking, or some respiratory-tract infections, such as sinusitis and bronchiectasis.

There are also a few conditions that affect the esophagus. Stress, muscular spasm, or dysfunction of the upper esophageal sphincter can all cause the sensation of having a lump in the throat. Difficulty in swallowing, or *dysphagia*, is a fairly common symptom with many possible causes, including stress, fungal infection or viral infection, and thyroid enlargement. However, it may also be the sign of a serious problem, such as myasthenia gravis, Parkinson's disease, narrowing of the esophagus, or throat or esophageal cancer.[1] Smoking and excessive alcohol consumption increase the risk of esophageal cancer. Esophageal varices, or enlarged veins in the esophagus, may develop as the result of liver problems. They can be dangerous because they tend to bleed.

Heartburn, or stomach acid reflux, occurs when material from the stomach backs up into the esophagus. Symptoms include a hot, burning, acidic sensation just behind the breastbone, and occasional regurgitation of warm, bitter fluid. This may interfere with sleep. As we saw in Chapter 1, there are many reasons for heartburn, including stress, smoking, and the consumption of alcohol or fatty foods. We also saw that many people use either antacids or the newer H2 blockers to try to quell heartburn, and how these drugs can do more harm than good.

Heartburn accompanied by chest pain, especially pain that radiates to the jaw, neck, or arm, or associated with other symptoms, such as cold sweats, nausea, or a squeezing sensation in the chest, may indicate a heart attack. If you experience such a combination of symptoms, do not wait for the discomfort to pass. *Seek medical attention immediately.*

According to William Perlow, M.D., gastroenterologist and attending physician at Mount Sinai Hospital in New York, there are ways to decide whether your heartburn and upset stomach warrant a visit to your physician:[2]

- If you regularly experience heartburn, try keeping a journal of the foods you eat and when you experience symptoms. Such a journal can help you become aware of any offending foods so you can eliminate or restrict your consumption of them.

- Remember that factors other than food can produce a sour stomach. The prime offenders are smoking, alcohol or caffeine consumption, and stress.

- Certain drugs can act as gastric irritants. Aspirin, Motrin, birth control pills, many antiarthritis drugs, and even some vitamins (such as those in the B complex) tend to increase your likelihood of suffering from a sour stomach.

Taking an over-the-counter antacid seldom gets to the source of your difficulty. It only offers immediate relief for heartburn associated with overindulgence. See your doctor if pain persists after taking an antacid, or if the pain is accompanied by fever or vomiting. Also see your doctor if the discomfort becomes chronic or the pain increases in intensity over a period of time, or if you experience weight loss, loss of appetite, nocturnal pain, or swallowing problems.

The esophagus passes through the diaphragm, the large muscle that separates the chest cavity from the abdominal cavity, through an opening called the *hiatus*. Sometimes, this opening becomes weakened because of injury, chronic constipation, obesity, pregnancy, smoking, or an inherited tendency towards weakness. When this happens, the juncture between the esophagus and the stomach can slide up into the chest cavity, creating a hiatus hernia. This is the most common form of hiatus hernia, occurring in about 75 percent of all cases. Sometimes, the junction remains in a normal position, but a pouch of stomach slides through the hiatus.

Symptoms of hiatus hernia include heartburn and belching. Bleeding from within the esophagus can lead to chronic blood loss, resulting in iron-deficiency anemia.

There are other minor conditions that affect this portion of the upper GI tract:

- Excessive belching is often caused by air swallowed as the result of eating too quickly.

- Hiccups occur when the diaphragm goes into repeated spasms, which forces bubbles of gas out of the stomach.

- The sensation of butterflies in the stomach come from anxiety, probably related to rapid beating of the abdominal aorta, the largest blood vessel in the body. This happens when adrenaline surges into the system, increasing both heart rate and blood pressure.

Stomach and Duodenum Disorders

These ailments include:

- *Peptic ulcer*, an open sore in the lining of the stomach or the duodenum

- *Gastritis,* irritation of the stomach lining

- *Miscellaneous disorders*, including achlorhydria, nonulcer dyspepsia, and nausea and vomiting of unknown origin

Peptic ulcer is a localized defect in the mucous membrane of the GI tract caused by exposure to stomach acid. The lesions are generally circular and about one inch in diameter. Usually, peptic ulcer occurs in the stomach or duodenum, although the jejunum, another section of the small intestine, may be occasionally involved. Chronic peptic ulcer becomes a prolonged disease, with alternating periods of more severe and less severe symptoms.

There are a number of factors that may contribute to ulcer development, including smoking, excessive caffeine or alcohol consumption, and a family history of ulcers. The use of certain drugs can also increase the risk of ulcer development, including aspirin and a family of painkillers called nonsteroidal anti-inflammatory drugs (NSAIDs), which are often prescribed for arthritis patients. About 30 percent of NSAID users are likely to develop a peptic ulcer. In addition, ulcer development is associated with a bacterium called *Helicobacter pylori* (see Chapter 4).

Symptoms of peptic ulcer include abdominal discomfort or pain, vomiting, nausea, heartburn, acid regurgitation, and constipation. Ulcer pain, which is localized, strikes both when the patient is hungry and about forty minutes after a meal. It is relieved by eating protein (which by itself acts as an antacid), taking antacid drugs, or vomiting. There may be weight loss, or there may be weight gain, as the patient consumes extra food to relieve his or her discomfort.

The use of antacids for the treatment of peptic ulcer can cause complications, especially since antacids must be used for a minimum of four weeks in such treatment.[3] For instance, if the kidneys do not work properly, the magnesium in some antacids can accumulate in the body, causing blood pressure problems and other difficulties. Magnesium can also interfere with the absorption of iron, the antibiotic tetracycline, and cimetidine (Tagamet). Calcium and aluminum, two other common antacid ingredients, can also cause these absorption problems. And as we saw in Chapter 1, the use of H2 blockers can result in other side effects. A better treatment for peptic ulcers uses probiotics (see Chapter 12).

Ulcers are a form of gastritis, a rather general term for an inflammation of the stomach lining. Gastritis can occur in response to acute physical stress, especially that produced by serious injuries or burns. It can also occur in a chronic form as the result of viral infection, Crohn's disease (see Chapter 3), or the use of drugs such as NSAIDs.

There are other types of stomach trouble. Achlorhydria is a syndrome in which the stomach acid is not acidic enough (a pH below 6.0). A chronic lack of hydrochloric acid can result in stomach cancer, increased risk of GI infections, or vitamin B_{12} deficiency.

Nonulcer dyspepsia is any form of painful, difficult, or disturbed digestion affecting either the upper or the lower part of the GI tract. It is the diagnosis doctors arrive at when tests and examinations have excluded organic disease such as peptic ulcer and cancer. Upper abdominal symptoms may come from delayed stomach emptying and chronic psychological stress. The best treatment consists of a low-fat diet eaten in smaller, more frequent meals, and the more extensive use of probiotics.

Nausea and vomiting of unknown cause can result from disturbances in the electrical rhythms of the stomach muscles. Just as in the heart, there is a pacemaker near the fundus that times and initiates the muscular contractions of the stomach.[4]

Liver, Gallbladder, and Pancreas Disorders

These ailments include:

- *Hepatitis*, inflammation of the liver
- *Cirrhosis*, chronic liver disease
- *Gallstones*, solid materials that form in the gallbladder or bile ducts
- *Cholecystitis*, inflammation of the gallbladder
- *Miscellaneous bile duct disorders*, including primary sclerosing cholangitis and primary biliary cirrhosis
- *Pancreatitis*, inflammation of the pancreas

Bile production is only one of the liver's many important functions, which include:

- The creation, breakdown, and storage of various substances used within the body
- The destruction of old red blood cells
- The disposal of various toxins, including alcohol and medication byproducts

This wide range of activities makes the liver vulnerable to a number of different disorders.

Hepatitis, or liver inflammation, can result from an infection by one of several different hepatitis viruses.

These viruses can be spread by contaminated food or blood. Hepatitis can also occur after infection with a variety of other organisms, including those that cause Epstein-Barr syndrome, tuberculosis, malaria, and syphilis. The intestinal disorders ulcerative colitis and Crohn's disease (see Chapter 3) can also cause it, as can a number of gallbladder disorders.

The signs of hepatitis include flulike symptoms, such as fever, fatigue, nausea, vomiting, diarrhea, and loss of appetite. These symptoms are followed by jaundice, a yellowing of the skin and eyes caused by bile buildup in the blood. Acute hepatitis may result in chronic hepatitis, which in turn may lead to cirrhosis.

Cirrhosis of the liver is a group of chronic diseases in which normal liver cells are damaged and replaced by scar tissue, thereby decreasing the amount of normal liver tissue. Chronic alcoholism is the most common cause of cirrhosis. Some people have genetic problems that cause metals such as copper or iron to accumulate in the liver, which can also lead to cirrhosis.

Symptoms of cirrhosis include fatigue, weakness, exhaustion, loss of appetite, nausea, diarrhea, lower extremity and abdominal swelling, jaundice, intense itching, dull mental functioning, and weight loss. However, the disease is sometimes "silent," with no early symptoms. It is treated through a combination of diet, prompt treatment of infections and bleeding, and avoidance of drugs and alcohol. In extreme cases, a liver transplant may be required.[5]

Gallstones are a major medical and economic problem in the United States. An estimated 22 million Americans, most of them women, suffer from gallstones. Gallstone surgery accounts for more than $2 billion in medical costs annually.

A person with gallstones may have a single large stone or a number of small ones. Once gallstones form, further stone formation is common. While there are "silent" stones, the main symptom is pain that occurs when a stone attempts to exit the gallbladder. Other symptoms include chills, fever, nausea, and vomiting. Jaundice develops when the flow of bile into the intestine is blocked. Symptoms are often triggered by the consumption of fatty foods. Gallstones can be removed surgically, dissolved through medication, or crushed by a shockwave treatment called lithotripsy.

Sometimes, the presence of gallstones can lead to cholecystitis, an infection or inflammation of the gallbladder. As in the case of gallstones, the main symptom is pain, generally following the consumption of fatty foods. Nausea and vomiting, belching, and jaundice may also occur. If removal of the stones does not cure the condition, the gallbladder may have to be removed.

Bile is carried by *bile ducts* within the liver, leading from the liver to the gallbladder, and leading from the gallbladder to the small intestine. These ducts can also become inflamed, which can lead to cirrhosis and blockage. Two conditions in which this occurs are primary sclerosing cholangitis (PSC) and primary biliary cirrhosis (PBC). The former most often occurs in young men, and is associated with inflammatory bowel disease (see Chapter 3). The latter most commonly affects middle-aged women, and is associated with autoimmune disorders such as scleroderma.

Pancreatitis is an inflammation of the pancreas, the large gland behind the stomach that secretes powerful digestive enzymes. (It also produces the blood-sugar regulators insulin and glucagon.) Inflammation occurs when those digestive enzymes attack the pancreatic tissues, leading to damage of the gland with bleeding and the formation of cysts or abscesses. When the patient experiences more than one attack, he or she is said to have relapsing pancreatitis. Acute relapsing pancreatitis is usually caused by gallstones, alcohol abuse, or certain drugs. About 80,000 cases of acute pancreatitis are diagnosed in the United States each year.

A mild steady pain in the upper abdomen that increases in severity and lasts for several days is characteristic of acute pancreatitis. The pain is:

- Constant

- Localized, radiating to the back

- Relieved by sitting or bending forward

- Accompanied by a swollen and tender abdomen

Other symptoms are nausea, vomiting, low-grade fever, increased pulse rate, jaundice, shortness of breath, dizziness, and pleurisy, an inflammation of the membranes lining the chest cavity.

A patient with acute pancreatitis is put on a strict fast, with nutrients supplied by intravenous fluids. A tube is placed through the nose into the stomach to remove gastric secretions. Surgery may be necessary if gallstones are present.

Chronic pancreatitis involves permanent damage to the organ, often from alcoholism. Total abstinence from alcohol is mandatory, but no other adequate treatment exists.[6]

The pancreas is also affected by cystic fibrosis, a genetic disease that affects mucus-producing glands located throughout the body, especially in the lung, intestine, and pancreas. The disorder causes a thick, sticky mucus to be produced. It is marked by fatty stools, poor weight gain despite good appetite, and chronic cough with frequent lung infections.

Some of these diseases discussed in this chapter are quite serious, and discussion of their treatment lies beyond the scope of this book. However, many of the more common disorders, such as heartburn and ulcers, respond well to the treatments we recommend in other chapters. In the next chapter, we will look at disorders that affect the lower GI tract.

CHAPTER 3

Problems in the Lower Digestive Tract

While heartburn and nausea are two of the most common symptoms of upper GI trouble, diarrhea and constipation are two of the most common symptoms of trouble in the lower GI tract. Most problems are not serious. However, some disorders, such as acute appendicitis, require immediate medical attention.

In this chapter, after a quick review of the organs and functions of the lower GI tract, we will look at the disorders that affect this part of the body. (For more information on the upper GI tract and its disorders, see Chapter 2. For information on a specific disorder or organ, contact the appropriate organization in Appendix A.)

ANATOMY AND FUNCTION OF THE LOWER GI TRACT

The lower GI tract includes most of the small intestine, also referred to as the small bowel; the large intestine, also referred to as the large bowel; and the anus (see

Figure 2.1). These organs are made of the same four types of tissue that make up most of the upper GI tract (see page 16).

Food passes from the stomach into the duodenum, the first part of the small intestine, which is considered to be part of the upper GI tract. The rest of the small intestine consists of the *jejunum*, which is from three to four feet in length, and the *ileum*, which is from six to seven feet long. In addition to the pancreatic juice and bile that enters the digestive tract at the duodenum, the intestinal walls themselves produce *intestinal juice*, which completes the digestive process. At this point, the proteins, carbohydrates, and fats in the original food have been reduced into nutrients: amino acids, simple sugars, fatty acids, and glycerol.

The small intestine has a vast absorptive surface, about the size of a doubles tennis court. That is because the inside of the small intestine consists of slender, fingerlike projections called *villi*. Most of the nutrients in the food are absorbed into the bloodstream from the villi in the small intestine.

The material that remains after the nutrients are absorbed passes from the small intestine into the large intestine, which consists of the *cecum*, the *colon*, the *rectum*, and the *anal canal*. Attached to the cecum, which receives food from the small intestine, is the *appendix*. The colon goes up, across, and down the abdomen before bending into the rectum. Accordingly, it is divided into the *ascending, transverse, descending*, and *sigmoid* (or S-shaped) portions. The colon is essentially a cylinder of varying widths, with the cecum being the widest and the sigmoid area the narrowest.

The large intestine absorbs water and various salts from the remaining material, which is formed into stool. The small plants and animals that live in a healthy human intestine, known collectively as the *gut flora*, produce vitamins and amino acids, which are also absorbed. The stool moves into the rectum, where pressure against the inner and outer *anal sphincters* triggers release through the anus.

DISORDERS AFFECTING THE LOWER GI TRACT

As we saw in Chapter 1, Americans spend billions of dollars annually on digestive aids of all sorts, including remedies for constipation and diarrhea. In this section, we will look at disorders that affect the lower GI tract. For information on the leaky gut syndrome, a disorder related to poor digestion, see Chapter 6.

Malabsorption and Intolerance Disorders

These ailments include:

- *Malabsorption syndrome*, any condition in which the intestine is unable to digest or absorb food

- *Celiac disease*, also known as gluten intolerance or nontropical sprue, a condition in which gluten, a protein found in grain, causes an abnormal chemical response in the bowel lining

- *Lactose intolerance*, an inability to digest dairy products

Malabsorption syndrome refers to any condition under which nutrients are poorly absorbed from the intestines. It can be caused by disease of the pancreas, gallbladder, or liver. It can also follow intestinal surgery or some of the other intestinal disorders described in this chapter. Symptoms include diarrhea, weakness, gas, weight loss, and bulky, foul-smelling stools that contain undigested fat.

One form of malabsorption, celiac disease, is caused by an intestinal allergy to gluten. This protein is found in wheat and rye, and to a lesser degree in barley and oats. Attacks are triggered by the consumption of bread, cakes, stuffings, or pasta, or of the gluten that is often added to such foods as soups, sauces, and ice cream. This leads to the poor absorption of these foodstuffs, with subsequent loss of weight, bloating, fatty stools, and, sometimes, diarrhea. There is damage to the intestinal mucous membrane, which includes loss of villi. An itchy rash called *dermatitis herpetiformis* (also known as Duhring's disease) may be associated with celiac disease. (For more information on food allergies, see "Testing for Food Allergies" on page 70 and *Hidden Food Allergies* in Appendix B.)

Elimination of gluten from the diet usually relieves symptoms, and confirms a diagnosis of celiac disease.[1] Sometimes, chicken or eggs must be eliminated, too. The use of probiotics may also bring relief (see Chapter 12).

Another form of malabsorption is called lactose intolerance. It is caused by a deficiency of lactase, the enzyme that digests lactose, which is a sugar found in milk and milk products. This deficiency leads to diarrhea, abdominal cramps, gas, and nausea whenever milk is consumed. Lactose intolerance occurs most often among Asians, African-Americans, and Native Americans. Treatment involves reducing the amount of milk in the diet and using commercial products containing lactase.

Diarrhea and Infectious Diseases

Diarrhea is a condition in which exceedingly loose bowel movements occur much more often than usual, and often results from many of the conditions described in this chapter. It can also be caused by stress, adverse drug reactions, or spoiled food. In addition, diarrhea can be caused by a synthetic fat called olestra (see "Why You Should Avoid Olestra" on page 34).

Diarrhea can also arise from infectious agents, such as those that sometimes afflict travelers, especially those traveling in areas where water supplies are not adequately treated. Traveler's diarrhea is often accompanied by abdominal cramps, fever, vomiting, or blood in the stool. It is most commonly viral in origin, but can involve bacteria such as *Escherichia coli* or those in the *Staphylococci* family. Parasites, including *Giardia lamblia*, *Entamoeba histolytica*, and *Cryptosporidium parvum*, can also cause this problem (see Chapter 8). You can prevent traveler's diarrhea by fortifying your intestines with probiotic bacteria (see Chapter 12). These bacteria, which can be taken in capsule form, can compete with disease-causing invaders.[2]

Obstructive Diseases and Disorders

These ailments include:

- *Polyps*, grapelike growths within the intestines
- *Intestinal obstruction*, a mechanical or physical blockage of the intestines
- *Cancer*, most commonly of the large intestine and especially of the rectum

Polyps occur most often in the large intestine. They either grow flat against the intestinal wall, or on little stalks. They usually cause no symptoms, although sometimes they may cause bleeding, cramps, or the passage of mucus. Often, the tendency to develop polyps runs in families. Some types of polyps may become cancerous, with the risk of malignancy increasing as the polyp increases in size.

Why You Should Avoid Olestra

Good taste, no calories: The food company that could offer the best of both worlds to dieters could reap a tremendous profit. That is why Proctor & Gamble spent more than $200 million in developing olestra (marketed under the trade name Olean), a fat substitute made from sugar and vegetable oil that is supposed to taste like the real thing. Because olestra's molecules are too large and tightly packed for digestive enzymes to break them down, this substance passes directly through the body. One of olestra's advantages for food manufacturers is that it survives the high heat necessary for fried snack foods such as potato chips.

However, olestra's possible side effects have made its use controversial. Among olestra's most widely reported side effects are those that affect the gastrointestinal system. They include nausea, bloating, diarrhea, and "anal leakage," in which there is uncontrolled elimination of a greasy liquid. The substance may also interfere with blood-thinning medications such as Coumadin.

In addition, olestra can deplete the body of valuable nutrients. The fat-soluble vitamins A, D, E, and K will dissolve in olestra, and thus be carried out of the body before they can be absorbed. P&G plans to add these vitamins to foods that contain the substance. There is also research showing that olestra may lower blood levels of some carotenoids, the large family of compounds that includes beta-carotene and lycopene, because these substances are also fat-soluble. The ingestion of carotenoids is associated with reduced rates of cancer, while low carotenoid levels in the blood are associated with heart disease and stroke. Carotenoids may also help prevent age-related macular degeneration, an eye disease that can result in blindness. It should also be noted that the widespread use of artificial fat may actually increase, rather than decrease, the incidence of obesity if people wind up eating more snack foods—which is what happened in the

1980s after a large number of products with artificial sweeteners entered the market.

The FDA requires that all foods containing olestra must be marked, and must carry a warning about its possible side effects. Obviously, the best way to avoid these side effects is to check the label carefully, and avoid foods containing this product.

Sources: M. Karstadt and S. Schmidt. Olestra: Procter's big gamble. *Nutrition Action Healthletter* 23(2):4–5, 1996; Olestra: Too good to be true? *Science News*, 27 January 1996; S. Meeker-Lowry. Greasing gluttony with olestra. *Food & Water Journal* 5(2):28–29, 1996.

There are a number of reasons why the intestines can become partially or completely obstructed, including paralysis of the intestinal muscles, surgical adhesions, intestinal hernias, twists or foreign objects in the intestines, severe constipation, and tumors or other masses. Symptoms include abdominal cramps, nausea and vomiting, weakness, bloating, and sometimes fever. A partial blockage may result in diarrhea, or no stools may be passed at all.

The incidence of colorectal cancer is second only to that of lung cancer in Western countries. It is linked to a diet that is low in fiber and high in fat (see Chapters 9 and 11), and there is some evidence that alcohol consumption may increase the risk.[3] Colorectal cancer often causes no symptoms in its early stages. Later symptoms include abdominal or rectal pain, a feeling of fullness, weight loss, and changes in bowel habits. The stools may contain dark-colored blood, as opposed to the bright-red blood that comes from hemorrhoids (see page 43). Early detection increases the chances of a full recovery. Small-intestine cancer occurs much more rarely, and is often related to an underlying disorder, such as Crohn's disease (see page 37).

Other Bowel Diseases and Disorders

These ailments include:

- *Constipation,* the infrequent, difficult, or inadequate passage of stool

- *Inflammatory bowel diseases,* including Crohn's disease, an inflammatory disease that most often affects the ileum or large intestine, and ulcerative colitis, a chronic inflammatory disease of the lining of the large intestine

- *Diverticular diseases,* including diverticulosis, a condition in which there are little sacs called diverticula in the wall of the large intestine, or diverticulitis, a condition in which diverticula become inflamed

- *Irritable bowel syndrome,* a disorder characterized by gas, abdominal pain, and diarrhea and/or constipation

- *Appendicitis,* an inflammation of the appendix

- *Ischemic bowel disease,* tissue damage due to insufficient blood supply to the intestine

The difficult passage of stools is known as constipation. It may occur in elderly or bedridden patients who do not move around much. This is called *atonic* constipation, or inactive colon. Constipation may also occur in nervous people who are prone to the effects of stress. This is called *spastic* constipation, or irritable colon. Constipation may also occur as a result of many of the conditions described in this chapter.

However, by far the most common cause of constipation is an inadequate amount of fiber in the diet and insufficient numbers of friendly bacteria to process that fiber. Once fiber enters the colon, bacteria digest it, adding bulk to the stool. In fact, half of the normal stool usually is made up of friendly bacteria. Increased stool bulk allows faster and easier passage of stool. This prevents constipation caused by the retention of dry, hard stool, also known as *dyschezia*. For more information on fiber and friendly bacteria, see Chapters 11 and 12.

Inflammatory bowel disease is actually a spectrum of overlapping symptoms that can be divided into two distinct disorders, Crohn's disease and ulcerative colitis. Between 1 and 2 million Americans suffer from these disorders, which are marked by episodes of acute disease that may be separated by years of symptom-free living. Inflammatory bowel disease is often linked to other inflammatory diseases, including arthritis and a number of skin conditions. Both Crohn's disease and ulcerative colitis are associated with an increased risk of cancer. They are usually treated with antibiotics, steroids, and/or surgery.

Crohn's disease, also known as regional enteritis, most often affects the ileum. However, it can affect any portion of the GI tract, from the mouth to the anus. Among the populations of Western industrialized countries, the occurrence of Crohn's disease is about five persons per 100,000. In the United States, it takes place more frequently, in about nine per 100,000 citizens. It is more common among Jews and among people with a family history of Crohn's disease.

Doctors are not sure what causes Crohn's disease. Researchers have examined immune system problems, infections, and poor diet as possible causes. However, there is no proof that any or all of these factors are involved.

Crohn's disease causes inflammation associated with ulceration, fissuring, and thickening of the intestinal wall. Benign tumors called granulomas develop within the intestinal lining. Frequently there are skip lesions, which are lesions separated by areas of normal bowel. Narrowing of the bowel may occur, and abnormal passages called fistulas may form. This can lead to intestinal obstruction and to the development of abscesses. There may be a long-term swelling affecting the ileum called Crohn's ileitis, or there may be proctitis involving the rectum (see page 43).

The symptoms of Crohn's disease include cramping pain, especially after eating; abdominal tenderness; nausea; diarrhea; general ill health; fever, chills, and weakness; and both appetite and weight loss. Patients with Crohn's disease are often depressed because of its chronic, long-lasting nature.[4] The addition of probiotics to the diet may ease the discomforts of this illness (see Chapter 12).

As its name indicates, ulcerative colitis is an inflammation of the lining of the large intestine. Its cause is unknown. Ulcerative colitis causes a general redness of the intestinal lining, with a lot of mucus and pus on the surface. Abscesses can develop, and the affected section of intestine often dilates and loses muscular tone. This disorder can lead to such serious complications as peritonitis (see page 44).

Early symptoms of ulcerative colitis include left-side pain that decreases after a bowel movement and attacks of bloody diarrhea. During acute attacks, the diarrhea becomes more frequent, and is accompanied by cramps, sweating, nausea, bloating, and fever.

Henry D. Janowitz, M.D., Clinical Professor of Medicine, Emeritus, at the Mount Sinai School of Medicine in New York, believes that the disorders connected with inflammatory bowel disease behave like infections. A form of paratuberculosis is suspected as the cause. This organism resembles the so-called slow viruses, in which symptoms develop years after the initial infection.[5] The use of probiotics may be useful.

Diverticulosis is a pouchlike bulging through the muscular layer of the large intestine, without any inflammation. It usually affects people age forty-five and above, and most often affects the sigmoid colon, which is the narrowest part of the large intestine. Some form of diverticulosis affects between 30 and 40 percent of all persons over age fifty.

Diverticula of the colon develop in areas of potential weakness as the result of the force exerted by the muscular layers of the intestine. This force is highest in the narrowest area of the colon, the sigmoid, where the waste contents are more solid than fluid. Because of constant pressure, the muscle wall thickens in the narrow areas and balloons out the thin inner and outer layers of the colon. Diverticulosis is most likely the result of the modern, highly refined, low-fiber diet common in industrialized nations. There is evidence that a lack of bulk in the stool causes the large intestine to spasm, putting pressure on the intestinal walls.[6]

Many patients with this condition have few symptoms except for occasional rectal bleeding, gas, and vague stomach distress. Other reasons for rectal bleeding, such as the presence of cancer and other bowel disease, must be ruled out. Treatment involves adding fiber to the diet, rest, a heating pad to relieve discomfort, and the use of probiotics.

Diverticulosis can lead to serious complications. One is perforation of the diverticula, which can lead to peritonitis (see page 44). Another is an inflammation of the diverticula, a condition known as diverticulitis. This condition is caused by fecal matter seeping through the thin-walled diverticula, which allows harmful bacteria to invade the tissues surrounding the colon. This leads to swelling and abscess formation. With repeated swelling, the opening of the colon narrows even more and sometimes becomes blocked. During an attack of diverticulitis, the patient will experience crampy pain, particularly in the lower abdomen, and fever.

Mild and moderate attacks of diverticulitis are treated with bedrest and antibiotics. Severe attacks require surgery. A colostomy, an opening between the colon and body surface, is created to rest the bowel for about six months. After this time, the colostomy is reversed.

However, there is another option besides antibiotics and surgery. The use of probiotics (see Chapter 12) can restock the large intestine with a friendly genus of bacteria known as *Bifidobacteria*. These organisms help the body in several ways:[7]

- They prevent harmful bacteria or yeasts from colonizing the intestine by competing for attachment sites and nutrients.

- They produce acids that make the intestine inhospitable for other, possibly harmful, bacteria.

- They inhibit bacteria that can alter chemicals called nitrites, which are known to be toxic and potentially carcinogenic.

- They manufacture essential B vitamins.

Irritable bowel syndrome (IBS) is a common, chronic problem of either the small or large intestine, or both. The ratio of women to men who are affected is more than two to one, and most patients are under the age of forty. People with IBS have a heightened perception of normal intestinal distention and contraction, which triggers disordered activity of the intestinal muscles.

The main symptoms of IBS are abdominal pain along with diarrhea and constipation, which sometimes alternate. The abdominal pain in IBS varies from mild to severe, is either dull or cramping in nature, and is usually situated in the lower abdomen or in the area around the navel. It is eased by defecation and the passage of gas. The diarrhea comes on very urgently, either upon rising, or during or after a meal. The constipation consists of hard and infrequent stools that require excessive straining.[8]

IBS is divided into subgroups based on differing groups of symptoms:

- Chronic or recurrent abdominal pain with an accompanying alteration of diarrhea and constipation, which is called spastic colon. This is the most common subgroup, and some authorities now restrict the definition of IBS to this symptom complex.

- Chronic painless diarrhea, which is called functional diarrhea.

- Chronic constipation without significant abdominal pain, which is called functional constipation.

- Chronic or recurrent abdominal pain without an accompanying alteration of bowel habit, which is called chronic functional abdominal pain.

IBS patients tend to suffer more from the effects of stress and emotional conflict more than other people. Acute psychological stress clearly affects bowel motility. IBS may also be linked to various forms of food intolerance (see page 31). The use of probiotics is quite helpful in reducing the extent and frequency of symptoms. For example, it has been verified that antibiotics can trigger the IBS,[9] probably because friendly bacteria ordinarily present in the intestines are greatly diminished by the killing effects of antibiotics.

Sometimes, small bits of food enter the appendix, which can then become inflamed, swollen, and infected. This condition is called appendicitis, and it can be life-threatening if the appendix bursts, releasing bacteria into the abdominal cavity (see page 44). The earliest symptom is pain that begins close to the navel and travels to the lower right abdomen, which becomes tender. Fever and nausea develop, and constipation sets in because digestion is disrupted. Appendicitis may be another disease that is related to a low-fiber diet, especially since it is uncommon in those parts of the world where high-fiber diets are eaten.[10]

Usually, appendicitis is treated by removing the appendix. Some doctors will even remove a healthy appendix while performing another operation, such as a hysterectomy, on the theory that a removed appendix cannot cause trouble. However, the appendix contains lymphatic tissue, and is an important part of the digestive system's immune defenses. Therefore, it should not be removed without cause. In some cases, even advanced cases of appendicitis have been treated with antibiotics instead of surgery.[11]

In atherosclerosis, fatty deposits gather on the walls of the arteries, which can cause the arteries to become narrow and stiff. This can occur in the aorta, the body's main artery, and its main branches. One of these main branches, the mesenteric artery, supplies blood to the large intestine. If this artery becomes clogged, sections of the large intestine can lose their blood supply, becoming *ischemic*. This condition is called ischemic bowel disease, and can threaten the survival of both the intestine and the patient unless artery-clearing treatment is administered as soon as possible.

Rectal and Anal Disorders

These ailments include:

- *Fistulas*, abnormal openings between the rectum and the skin

- *Fissures*, cracks in the lining of the anus

- *Hemorrhoids*, enlarged veins in the anal area
- *Proctitis*, irritation of the anal area

Crohn's disease, diverticulitis, abscesses, and other disorders may lead to the development of an anal fistula, an opening from the anus to the surrounding skin. Fistulas are removed surgically.

An anal fissure is a tear or ulcer in the last inch of the rectum, which is known as the anal canal. Fissures, which are believed to develop due to laceration by a large or hard stool, cause pain upon defecation and rectal bleeding. Often, they respond to the use of laxatives and glycerin suppositories that allow the area to heal without further injury. If these measures fail, surgery is needed.

Hemorrhoids are the most common cause of rectal bleeding, and are the most common rectal disorder. Hemorrhoids, or piles, are varicose veins at the beginning of the anal canal, in the case of *internal hemorrhoids*, or at the anal opening, in the case of *external hemorrhoids*. They are often complicated by inflammation, clotting, and bleeding. They may result in pain, itching, or the passage of mucus upon defecation.

Several factors may combine to favor the development of hemorrhoids. They include lack of exercise, chronic intestinal disturbances, weakness of the connective tissue within the rectum, chronic inflammation in the anal area, overuse of laxatives, colon tumors, and poor blood circulation in the anal area.[12]

Hemorrhoids are often treated with stool-softeners to correct constipation and straining. Severe cases may require surgery. The best way to keep them from recurring—or to avoid them in the first place—is to eat a high-fiber diet and drink plenty of water (see Chapter 11).

Proctitis, an inflammation of the rectum and anal area, is associated with Crohn's disease, a variety of sexually transmitted diseases, and radiation therapy. Symptoms include pain and the passage of blood or mucus. Treatment consists of sitz baths, topical anesthetics, and, if a specific disease-causing organism is present, antibiotics.

Abdominal Cavity Disorders

These ailments include:

- *Peritonitis*, irritation of the lining of the abdominal cavity

- *Hernia*, an abnormal protrusion of the intestine or other organs through an opening in the abdominal wall

Peritonitis usually occurs when an intestinal disorder, such as diverticulitis, causes the GI tract to perforate and release its contents into the abdominal cavity. In such cases, the peritoneum, the membrane that covers all the abdominal organs, becomes inflamed. (Some disorders of the female reproductive system, such as a ruptured ectopic pregnancy, can also result in peritonitis.) Treatment includes giving the patient nutrients and fluid intravenously, and prescribing antibiotics. The condition can be life-threatening if not dealt with promptly.

We discussed hiatus hernia, in which part of the stomach slides up through the diaphragm, in Chapter 2. But hernias can occur elsewhere. The most common form of intestinal hernia is the inguinal hernia, in which a loop of intestine makes it way into the scrotum. This can be dangerous if the loop loses its blood supply and becomes strangulated, causing an intestinal blockage. Surgery corrects the problem.

As we have seen in Chapters 2 and 3, the GI tract is prone to a number of disorders. No wonder people develop indigestion! Now it is time to take a closer look at some of the more common disorders and how they can be treated. In the next chapter, we will take a closer look at ulcers.

CHAPTER 4

Fighting the Bacteria That Cause Ulcers

U lcers are among the most common digestive disorders. Doctors estimate that more than 13 million Americans are or have been victims of ulcers. Another 140 million or so people worldwide suffer with ulcers. Finding an effective way to deal with this affliction would go a long way to solving the problem of indigestion.

The idea that a bacterial infection could be linked to gastric ulcers has long been the subject of debate among medical scientists. That idea has been proven correct. Scientists now know that a common bacterium, *Helicobacter pylori* (previously called *Campylobacter pylori*), lies behind the development of most ulcers in the stomach and duodenum. Moreover, it may be possible to use friendly bacteria to compete with *H. pylori* and starve it out of existence.

In this chapter, we will first take a closer look at ulcers and how they were treated using the old conventional methods. We will then discuss the research that has been done on *H. pylori* and the role of probiotics in treating infections caused by this bacterium.

LESS STRESS, BLAND DIET:
THE OLD ULCER TREATMENT

As we explained in Chapter 2, a peptic ulcer is an eroded spot in the lining of the stomach (*gastric ulcer*) or
duodeum (*duodenal ulcer*). An ulcer occurs when the mucus produced by the digestive system fails to protect the
delicate lining from both stomach acid and *pepsin*, an
enzyme that speeds up the breakdown of protein. In es-
sence, the stomach starts to digest itself. Chronic ulcers
produce a gnawing pain in the upper abdomen frequently accompanied by the sensation of burning, belching, and nausea, especially when the stomach is empty
or after a fatty meal is consumed.

Ulcers had been thought to be caused by a number
of factors. They include excess stomach acid, loss of mucous membrane, overabundant stress, inherited defects,
and the patient's use of certain prescription and over-
the-counter drugs, such as aspirin and other painkillers.

Old treatment procedures used antacids or H2 blockers (see Chapter 1) and other drugs to control the symptoms. The patient was taught to eat many small meals
made up of nonirritating foods. And since ulcers had
usually been associated with stress, doctors usually recommended that patients practice some form of stress reduction.

ULCERS CONSIDERED AS A
BACTERIAL INFECTION

In the early 1980s, two Australian researchers, gastroenterologist Barry J. Marshall, M.D., and pathologist J.
Robin Warren, M.D., Ph.D., published research that
would eventually overturn what had been conventional
ulcer treatment. They claimed that a bacterium, *Helicobacter pylori*, was responsible for gastritis and ulcers

among their patients.[1,2] As part of their proof, they swallowed *H. pylori* and produced the unpleasant symptoms of gastritis and peptic ulcer in themselves.[3]

In this section, we will explain how the Marshall and Warren studies introduced scientists to a new theory of ulcer formation, and how this theory has been confirmed by other researchers.

Australian Studies Point the Way

Dr. Marshall and Dr. Warren did their initial studies in a hospital near Perth, on Australia's west coast. The first gastritis patient they successfully treated was a fifty-four-year-old woman who had suffered from digestive problems for twenty years. Her pain was so severe that doctors kept admitting her to the hospital's coronary care unit to rule out heart attack.

Dr. Marshall discovered that the woman's stomach was infected with *H. pylori*. She was treated with bismuth compound, a stomach soother, and a penicillin-type antibiotic called amoxicillin. A month later, a biopsy showed that her stomach was healing, and that she was secreting more gastric mucus. The infection did not return, and the patient's gastritis healed completely.

The two researchers went on to find that more than 93 percent of all patients who had duodenal ulcer with associated gastritis were infected with *H. pylori*. This was later confirmed worldwide in other industrialized countries. Moreover, according to Dr. Marshall, about 90 percent of patients with gastric cancer had infections, probably without symptoms, during the preceding twenty years. The link between *H. pylori* and cancer is still being studied,[4] although at least one study shows that people with gastric ulcers do run a higher risk of stomach cancer.[5]

With the isolation of *H. pylori*, the floodgates opened

for new areas of gastric disease research. Medical science now knows that *H. pylori* is responsible for most cases of chronic nonspecific gastritis, gastric ulcers, and duodenal ulcers. It is commonly found among people without any gastric symptoms in the United States, and is endemic in the populations of some developing nations, too.

H. pylori is communicable. According to Dr. Marshall, about half of his patients with *H. pylori* infections have spouses who are infected. He also says that about 20 percent of all patients with this infection carry the bacteria in their dental plaque.[6] Scientists are studying the possibility that flies spread *H. pylori* by carrying it on their bodies. In addition, dogs and cats are infected by other members of the *Helicobacter* family, which may be transferred to humans. This is especially true of children who do not wash their hands before they eat after playing with pets.

H. pylori is the only bacteria known to live in the stomach's very acidic environment. It adheres to the stomach's mucus-secreting cells and produces enzymes that allow it to reduce the acidity in the immediate area. The organism also decreases mucus production. Some studies have shown that when healthy volunteers ingest live cultures of *H. pylori,* many develop gastritis with symptoms that include pain, bloating, and nausea. The bacteria appear to digest the mucus layer, causing it to become thin and runny. Sometimes, the entire protective lining becomes eroded. This allows gastric acid and pepsin to come into direct contact with the unprotected cells of the stomach wall.

Despite the evidence, the manufacturers of the most widely prescribed ulcer treatments disregard the *H. pylori* information. Their concern is understandable, since sales of H2 blockers have tapered off since this information came to light.[7] While ulcers sometimes heal after a patient takes an H2 blocker, the problem often recurs.

Other Studies Support the *H. Pylori* Findings

At the Baylor College of Medicine in Texas, David Graham, M.D., and his colleagues studied 109 ulcer patients who had been randomly assigned to receive either Zantac alone or Zantac in combination with two antibiotics, tetracycline and metronidazole, plus an over-the-counter upset stomach remedy. The researchers found that 95 percent of all gastric ulcer patients on the multidrug regimen had no recurrences in the following two years. But only 12 percent of those who received Zantac by itself were ulcer-free in that period. Among patients with duodenal ulcers, the figures were 74 percent and 13 percent, respectively. Daniel Hollander, M.D., professor of gastroenterology at the University of California at Irvine, says the Graham findings "show you can prevent recurrence of ulcers if you eradicate *H. pylori*."[8] European research has shown similar results.[9]

Many other studies support the link between *H. pylori* and gastrointestinal disorders, because they have shown that ulcers and inflammation disappeared when the infection is treated and eliminated. In some studies, complete healing was reported in all gastritis patients upon elimination of the infection.

An important study, conducted by an independent panel convened by the National Institutes of Health (NIH), forced the medical community to rethink the old ulcer treatment. In its statement, the NIH panel said: "Ulcer patients with *H. pylori* infection require treatment with antimicrobial agents in addition to antisecretory drugs." Such a statement from the NIH, a governmental body, essentially put the government's stamp of approval on the *H. pylori* theory of gastric disease. This represented "an important sea change" in ulcer treatment policy, according to one panel member.[10]

Research on *H. pylori* continues. Scientists have now unscrambled the bacterium's genetic code, and this information will provide a deeper understanding of how the organism behaves and how it can be fought.[11]

PROBIOTICS AND ULCER TREATMENT

If ulcers are caused by an infection, why not just prescribe antibiotics? That would seem to be the simple answer, but as in many areas of medicine, the situation is not as simple as it appears. The problem is drug resistance, in which surviving germs are less and less likely to be affected by a given medication (see "The Dangers of Antibiotics" and *When Antibiotics Fail* in Appendix B). This could happen to antibiotic-based ulcer treatment. Gastroenterologist John H. Walsh, M.D., of UCLA warns that *H. pylori* could become resistant to antibiotics: "These antibiotics frequently cause side effects. And patients will become reinfected and develop ulcers again."[12]

One way to avoid drug resistance is to "seed" parts of the body with friendly, probiotic bacteria such as *Lactobacillus acidophilus*, *Bifidobacteria bifidum*, and *Bifidobacteria longum* (see Chapter 12). These bacteria have been shown to kill *H. pylori*.[13]

Harmful organisms such as *H. pylori* must attain certain population densities in the body before they can successfully invade the body's tissues. The presence of probiotic bacteria stops harmful bacteria from growing and spreading.[14] These good bacteria do that in several ways:[15]

• They take up living space in the gastrointestinal tract, thus offering no growing room for bad bacteria.

The Dangers of Antibiotics

In 1928, Alexander Fleming, M.D., the man who discovered penicillin, warned against using his miracle drug for every imaginable ill. Dr. Fleming recognized that penicillin did not kill all bacteria, and that survivors would likely resist subsequent doses of the drug. Sadly, Dr. Fleming's warnings have not been heeded. Antibiotics have been overused, leading to a situation called *antibiotic resistance.* This has come about for several reasons. Antibiotics have been overprescribed in cases of human illness, especially in the use of broad-spectrum drugs that kill many different types of germs. Antibiotics have also been overused through such agricultural practices as the addition of drugs to animal feed. Most of the world's mammals are now plagued by a whole new order of infections that were rare before the antibiotic era. In the words of biologist and toxicologist Marc Lappe', Ph.D.: "This is the weakness of our century—an uncritical acceptance of technological breakthroughs as . . . free from harmful side effects."[1]

Russia and other countries of the former Soviet Union present a frightening example of antibiotic use run rampant. A lack of infection control—American doctors were stunned to find that Russian surgeons did not wash hands between patients—and a huge black market in self-prescribed antibiotics have led to fatal epidemics of diseases, such as typhoid, that are easily treated in the West. Moreover, while many of these conditions existed during the Soviet era, the economic and social chaos unleashed by the USSR's breakup has only made matters worse. As a result of these abuses, many antibiotics, inclusing ciproflexacin and doxycycline, are now totally ineffective through overuse.[2]

Similar situations exist, in lesser degrees, in almost all industrialized countries. There are now drug-resistant strains of tuberculosis and gonorrhea, diseases once easily cured with antibiotics, and doctors must use second- or even third-generation antibiotics to treat a number of other bacterial diseases. In hospitals, the incidence of *nosocomial* infections, or infections unrelated to the patient's original condition, are rising at an alarming rate. These infections appear to be linked to the development of resistant strains of microbes within the hospital environment itself. Ironically, the array of lifesaving equipment so commonly used in modern medicine increases the risk of nosocomial infection. Devices such as breathing tubes and catheters introduce foreign material into the body, thus providing new pathways for germs. In addition, medications often provoke allergic reactions in sensitive individuals, ranging from rashes to shock, and any number of side effects, some of them quite severe.

How did this happen? At the end of World War II, other scientists took up Dr. Fleming's research, purifying penicillin and discovering its chemical composition. This gave rise to the mass production of antibiotics, and to a generation of doctors trained in their use. Drugs became the standard treatment for infection, and most people lost touch with traditional therapies.

As microbes have become more and more resistant, drug companies try to keep one step ahead of them by introducing new drugs at a rate of five to ten a year.[3] This is not a permanent solution: We must slow the rate of antibiotic use. In Sweden, for example, antibiotics are not routinely used in animal feed, and Swedish doctors prescribe narrow-spectrum drugs only after lab tests have determined exactly which microbe is responsible for a patient's illness. Eventually, we must all return to what one alternative-health writer calls a "common-sense approach" of initially waiting for the body to rally its own defenses before intervening with natural treatments, such as herbal or homeopathic remedies. In the meantime, if you must use an antibiotic, be sure to take the entire supply of pills, along with olive-leaf extract and 2 to 3 grams a day of vitamin C to enhance the drug's effectiveness, and use probiotic supplements to protect your digestive system.[4]

- They absorb a vast majority of the available nutrients, which deprives bad bacteria of nourishment.

- Many of them produce substances that are toxic to ulcer-forming bacteria.

- They encourage the body's immune system to fight these invaders.

Taken in supplement form (see Appendix C), probiotics provide a means of overcoming the dangers inherent in the overuse of antibiotics. This is especially important in dealing with illnesses of the digestive system, since antibiotics often disrupt the friendly bacteria normally found in the human intestines. The consumption of yogurt, which contains probiotic bacteria, is another way of keeping disease-causing microbes at bay (see Chapter 10). In addition, research shows a link between a low-fiber diet and an increased incidence of duodenal ulcer,[16] so adding fiber to the diet may help prevent ulcer formation. (For more information on fiber, see Chapter 11.) If ulcers do develop, antibiotics should be taken for as short a time as possible. It is important to use probiotic supplements *along with* any prescribed antibiotics, and to keep taking the supplements after drug treatment ends. That allows the antibiotics to perform their function while minimizing the harm done to the digestive system overall.

The discovery of *H. pylori* and its link to stomach disorders has revolutionized the treatment of gastric disease. However, antibiotics are not the ultimate answer. Probiotics consumption is the best defense against ulcers, insuring that abundant amounts of beneficial microbes will be present in the intestines. In the next chapter, we will explain the link between bad bacteria and intestinal dysfunction.

CHAPTER 5

How Bad Bacteria Can Harm the Intestines

Since the nineteenth century, when medical scientists first identified the links between indigestion and chronic illness, it has been recognized that what happens in the intestines can have far-reaching effects on what happens in the body as a whole. This has included an awareness that intestinal bacteria, whether beneficial or harmful, determine a person's digestive health. Normally, the relationship between the body and the intestinal bacteria is one of eu-symbiosis, or *eubiosis*, which means there is a balanced and positive effect on health. When the good and bad bacteria in the intestines become unbalanced, the result is a state known as dys-symbiosis, or *dysbiosis*.

In this chapter, we will first explain how dysbiosis can harm health. We will then discuss how dysbiosis affects both the small and large intestines, and how you can avoid or correct this problem.

THE SIGNIFICANCE OF INTESTINAL DYSBIOSIS

Elie Metchnikoff, a Russian scientist working at the turn of the twentieth century, popularized the concept of dysbiosis. He concluded that the bacterial putrefaction of food produced toxic substances known as *amines*, which he thought caused degenerative disease. Metchnikoff also popularized the idea that ingestion of foods containing live cultures of good microbes such as the *Lactobacilli* could prolong life by decreasing intestinal putrefaction.[1] The notion that dysbiosis influences the development of inflammatory diseases and cancer has received considerable support in the laboratory. But the mechanisms involved are far more diverse than Metchnikoff ever imagined.

The entire digestive system, from mouth to anus, is home to billions of microbes. These include yeasts and a wide variety of bacteria, with different organisms living in different parts of the system. When a state of eubiosis exists, most of the organisms are the good, healthy kind. Any bad microbes, if present, are not capable of spreading too rapidly or producing overwhelming amounts of toxins. They are kept in check by the good microbes, which dominate the available food supply and produce chemicals that inhibit the growth of undesirable organisms.

However, if large numbers of bad microbes are introduced into the system, or if the amount of good microbes is reduced, an imbalance is created that favors the bad organisms. This imbalance hinders digestion by reducing the effectiveness of various digestive secretions and by damaging the intestinal villi, among other ill effects. More than that, imbalance, or dysbiosis, allows the bad microbes to attack the body's immune system. If the immune system is weak—as the result of stress, poor nutrition, or exposure to toxins—the bad organisms can escape from the intestines into the bloodstream. Thus, harmful intestinal microbes can promote disease in other parts of the body.

THE EFFECTS OF SMALL INTESTINE DYSBIOSIS

The most common reason for small intestine dysbiosis is the overgrowth of disease-producing bacteria in the *Coccobacilli* and *Streptococci* families.[2,3] The presence of parasites may also predispose a person to bacterial overgrowth[4] (see Chapter 8). Bacteria can multiply for several other reasons:[5]

- Gastric hypochlorhydria, or lack of stomach acid
- Stasis, or failure of food to move normally through the intestines
- Obstruction due to either a narrowing of the intestinal opening or the presence of abnormal passages called fistulas
- Immune deficiency
- Malnutrition

The overgrowth of bad bacteria damages the small intestine in a variety of ways. Much of the damage resulting from small bowel dysbiosis results from the action of protein-destroying enzymes called *proteases* that are produced by the bacteria. The proteases damage the mucous membrane and cause malabsorption, or the inability of the intestine to absorb vital nutrients. Bacterial consumption of vitamin B_{12} lowers blood levels of this vitamin, which may result in a vitamin deficiency and subsequent symptoms. Bile salts are also degraded.[6]

O. Hunter, M.D., and his colleagues discovered that diarrhea, cramps, and specific food intolerances are related to the presence of abnormal organisms in the stool.[7-9] In Crohn's disease, a condition associated with damage to the intestinal wall, patients who suffer from diarrhea and show signs of malabsorption have an exaggerated immune system response to organisms normally found in the stool. The "bad" bacteria lead these people to become allergic to their own stools.[10] Some bacterial infections of the small bowel increase intestinal permeability, often referred to as the leaky gut syndrome (see Chapter 6).[11] Presence of the leaky gut syndrome in patients with active Crohn's disease and in members of their immediate families suggests the existence of a pre-existing abnormality that allows an exaggerated immune system response to normal stools.[12] (For more information on Crohn's disease, see Chapter 2.)

Small bowel dysbiosis has also been found to cause disease beyond the intestines. Studies show that animals suffer liver damage from the poisons given off by bad bacteria. The same difficulties can potentially arise in human beings.[13] In addition, gastroenterologist and dermatologist George Ionescu, M.D., and his colleagues discovered that atopic eczema, a skin disorder, was associated with dysbiosis and malabsorption in a majority of patients who suffered such intestinal conditions.[14,15]

THE EFFECTS OF LARGE INTESTINE DYSBIOSIS

Generally, large bowel dysbiosis is associated with a diet that is high in meat and fat, and low in fiber. Like small bowel dysbiosis, it can produce a number of adverse effects.

As we saw at the beginning of the chapter, Elie Metchnikoff was the first person to see the connection between poor digestion and amines, toxic substances linked to degenerative diseases. Scientists have since discovered a number of amines, including histamine, which you may know as a chemical involved in allergic reactions. Amines are formed from amino acids, the building blocks of proteins, by bad bacteria in the large intestine. Because blood from the large intestine first passes into the liver, these amines become absorbed into the liver for circulation through the portal system, a network of veins that connects the liver with the stomach, intestines, spleen, pancreas, and gallbladder. When liver cirrhosis is present, the amines reach the body's general blood circulation. Thus, they contribute to the brain defects and low blood pressure that are frequently associated with liver failure.[16]

Eating a high-meat diet can also result in chemical reactions that lead to cancer. Some species of bad intestinal bacteria produce an enzyme that turns urea, a normal protein digestion byproduct, into ammonia, which is highly alkaline and thus raises stool pH. Medical science now recognizes that a relatively high stool pH is associated with a higher incidence of colon cancer.[17] Similar types of harmful microorganisms produce an enzyme that degrades the amino acid tryptophan into phenols, which are carcinogenic.[18]

Other enzymes produced by bad intestinal bacteria degrade what are called conjugated estrogens, a form of the main female sex hormone that relieves the symptoms of menopause, producing *deconjugated estrogens*. Women (and men) who eat a high-fat, low-fiber diet show increased levels of deconjugated estrogens in the stool. That, in turn, raises estrogen levels in the blood and urine. The circulation of deconjugated estrogens possibly contributes to the development of breast and prostate cancer.[19]

Bile acids can also be deconjugated by bad intestinal bacteria. Such deconjugated bile acids are poisonous to the mucous membrane that lines the colon, and usually produce diarrhea. Deconjugated bile acids and their byproducts are thought to contribute to the development of colon cancer[20] and ulcerative colitis.[21]

In addition, bad intestinal bacteria reduce primary bile acids to secondary bile acids, which do not stimulate digestion as efficiently as primary acids. Furthermore, secondary bile acids are not absorbed as readily and are more likely to contribute to colon cancer.

HOW TO AVOID OR CORRECT DYSBIOSIS

As we have said, the modern Western diet, with its emphasis on refined sugars and fats, meat, and processed foods, is an important factor in the development of dysbiosis. Decreases in fiber and fluid consumption slow down the transport of stool through the large intestine. That allows increased time for putrefaction and leads to an increase in the number of harmful microbes.

Another important factor is the overuse of antibiotics (see "The Dangers of Antibiotics" on page 53). Such abuse not only leads to the development of disease-producing bacteria that are drug resistant, but antibiotics also kill the friendly bacteria the body needs for proper digestion.

It is important to remember that dysbiosis is a clinical concept, not a disease. Exploring this concept calls for an method of investigation that goes beyond the conventional medical practice of labeling a disease and thinking that the label itself causes the symptoms. Such an approach may be appropriate when dealing with an acute infection, such as strep throat. But the practice of labeling chronic disease in this manner leads to the erroneous practice of treating the label with a drug or another type of stopgap therapy to suppress the patient's immediate discomforts, while not necessarily curing the disease.[22]

Treatment for dysbiosis must go beyond labels. As wholistic practitioner Sidney Baker, M.D., puts it, "Each of us is unique with special requirements which, if unmet, cause or worsen chronic illness. Each of us is indivisible, and therefore the integration of various systems and organs may be as important in health as the function of any particular organ."[23] Such an approach requires a willingness to find each patient's optimum nutrition needs, and to identify the allergens and toxins that can produce or aggravate dysbiosis. It also requires the active participation of the patient, who must make wise decisions about everyday living, with the doctor serving as a consultant and guide.

Dysbiosis can be a difficult condition to correct, requiring a long-term approach and strict compliance by the patient. Such an approach includes:

- Eliminating simple sugars from the diet
- Avoiding food additives such as monosodium glutamate, caffeine, and artificial sweetners[24]
- Reducing meat consumption to just one meal a week or less
- Increasing fluid and fiber intake in order to normalize stool transit time (see Chapter 11)
- Using probiotic food supplements (see Chapter 12 and Appendix C) to recolonize the intestinal tract with good bacteria
- Avoiding contact, to the extent possible, with disease-producing germs
- Avoiding, if at all possible, the use of antibiotics

  Other recommended actions include:
- Supplementing the diet with vitamins, minerals, and essential fatty acids
- Using stress reduction measures, such as meditation
- Increasing the nightly hours of sleep
- Exercising at least thirty minutes each day
- Getting more sunlight exposure, with sunblock protection

We would also recommend the Mediterranean diet (see Chapter 9), which emphasizes high-fiber, low-fat foods. This includes an abundance of fresh fruits and vegetables, which are good sources of enzymes that help prevent dysbiosis.

Dysbiosis can create havoc in both the small and large intestines, upsetting digestion and leading to disease in other parts of the body. A long-term program of diet, exercise, and rest, plus supplementation with probiotics and other important substances, can overcome dysbiosis. In the next chapter, we will discuss the leaky gut syndrome.

CHAPTER 6

Poor Digestion and the Leaky Gut Syndrome

Digestion is a process by which food—what the body might consider to be a "foreign" substance—is changed into substances that the body's cells can absorb. When digestion is faulty, the body is faced with the burden of sorting out *self*, or safe substances, from *nonself*, or unsafe substances. Hypersensitivity reactions, allergies, and other adverse responses to foods and other substances may, therefore, be related to a problem present in the digestive system, whether the symptoms are digestive in nature or not. That includes conditions such as hives, asthma, congestion, and fatigue.

Over time, disruptions of the gastrointestinal immune system can lead to hyperpermeability of the intestines, a situation in which substances other than nutrients pass with relative ease through the intestinal walls and into the circulatory system. This is called the leaky gut syndrome.

The leaky gut syndrome is a factor in dysbiosis of either the large or small intestine (see Chapter 5). Actually, this syndrome is the source of a great deal of disease. In this chapter, we will first discuss the nature of the leaky gut syndrome. We will then show you what specific conditions are associated with it, and how it can be treated.

THE NATURE OF THE LEAKY GUT SYNDROME

Immune system damage can result from frequent and chronic indigestion. Many people take chronic indigestion too lightly, and use large amounts of antacids to counteract digestive upsets. While antacids may provide temporary relief, they do not address the real problem, and eventually the immune system may not respond as well as it should.

Indigestion, and the subsequent malabsorption of vital nutrients, is not the only reason for immune-system malfunction. Exposures to toxic metals or polluting chemicals, or the presence of viral, fungal, or parasitic infections, are among the other factors that can damage the body's defenses. Stress is another important factor.

A poor immune response may cause the immune system to not be as sensitive as it should be to foreign substances, a condition that can lead to frequent bouts of illness. Or, conversely, a poor immune response can cause the body to become overly sensitive, or allergic, to substances in the diet or the environment, or even to its own tissues. Under such circumstances, the intestinal walls become too permeable, with the result that disease-causing microbes and other harmful substances can enter the body. Ordinarily, the intestinal lining restricts the passage of noxious elements, a characteristic referred to as the *barrier function* of the lining. In the leaky gut syndrome, this barrier function fails.

The most common causes of the leaky gut syndrome damage are infections,[1-4] alcohol,[5,6] and the routine use of almost any of the nonsteroidal anti-inflammatory drugs (NSAIDs).[7-9] Other causes include certain types of drugs,[10-12] such as those used in cancer chemotherapy, and a reduction in the intestinal oxygen supply as the result of either open-heart surgery or shock.[13,14] There is evidence that the leaky gut syndrome affects a diverse group of people, including smokers, diabetics, and long-distance runners.[15]

CLINICAL CONDITIONS ASSOCIATED WITH THE LEAKY GUT SYNDROME

While the leaky gut syndrome itself is not a disease, a number of serious health problems are associated with it. In the following conditions, this connection has been verified:

- Various intestinal diseases,[16-21] such as inflammatory bowel disease, Crohn's disease, ulcerative colitis, celiac disease, and intestinal infections

- Various chronic arthritic diseases,[22-27] such as inflammatory joint disease

- Various skin conditions, such as acne, psoriasis, and dermatitis herpetiformis[28-31]

- Diseases triggered by food allergy or specific food intolerance, including eczema, urticaria, and irritable bowel syndrome[32-40]

- Chronic fatigue and immune dysfunction syndrome (see Chapter 12); Dr. Leo Galland, who has worked with many leaky gut syndrome patients, thinks that the syndrome plays a role in 70 percent of all chronic fatigue cases[41]

- Chronic hepatitis[42]

- Chronic pancreatitis[43,44] and pancreatic cancer

- Multiple chemical sensitivities and environmental illness
- Autism and childhood hyperactivity
- Alcoholism

Other diseases that are thought to be associated with the leaky gut syndrome include:

- AIDS[45-47]
- Cystic fibrosis[48]
- Schizophrenia
- Giardiasis, a parasitic infestation (see Chapter 8)

Doctors also think there is a connection between the syndrome and the aging process.

Symptoms associated with the leaky gut syndrome include:

- Fatigue and malaise
- Joint and muscle pain
- Fever of unknown origin
- Food intolerances
- Abdominal pain and distention
- Diarrhea
- Skin rashes
- Problems in mental functioning
- Shortness of breath and poor exercise tolerance

TREATMENT STRATEGIES FOR THE LEAKY GUT SYNDROME

As in the case of intestinal dysbiosis (Chapter 5), treatment of the leaky gut syndrome requires rejection of the old disease- and drug-oriented approach to illness. Instead, it requires the acknowledgment that each patient is unique, with a unique set of nutritional requirements and sensitivities. Such an approach gives each patient what he or she needs without focusing on labeling the illness.[49]

Wholistic physicians concentrate on the connections among intestinal inflammation, increased gut permeability, and autoimmune disease. Monitoring intestinal permeability in patients with the leaky gut syndrome is an important part of treatment, especially since there are safe and inexpensive methods of doing so. Such monitoring can help improve a patient's outcome.[50] Maintaining a close control over diet, especially in patients with food allergies, is another vital aspect of treatment. (For more information on food allergies, see "Testing for Food Allergies" on page 70 and *Hidden Food Allergies* in Appendix B.)

A number of substances are used in wholistic treatment of the leaky gut syndrome:

- *Cromolyn sodium* inhibits an allergic response to food allergens by affecting histamine-sensitive cells called mast cells. Quercitin, a natural bioflavonoid, also stabilizes mast cells.

- *Glutamine*, an amino acid, prevents and reverses damage to the intestinal mucous membrane caused by various noxious agents (see *The Ultimate Nutrient: Glutamine* in Appendix B).

- *Ginkgo biloba extract*, a long-used herbal remedy, prevents mucous membrane damage caused by loss of blood flow. It may also have an antiallergy effect and is an important antioxidant.

- *Butyric acid*, a fatty acid produced by bacteria in the lower intestines as a byproduct of fiber fermentation,

Testing for Food Allergies

Food allergies occur when the immune system overreacts to a specific food by producing antibodies, substances responsible for the discomforts associated with allergies. Food allergies cause not only gastrointestinal symptoms, including nausea, diarrhea, constipation, and flatulence, but a whole host of other symptoms as well, including headaches, eye and ear problems, runny or stuffy nose, heart palpitations, urinary infections, arthritis, hives, fatigue, and depression. In some cases, the reaction is immediate, such as hives that appear after a meal of shellfish. In others, the reaction is delayed for hours, even days. A delayed reaction makes it difficult to know exactly which food is causing the problem, or if a food allergy is responsible in the first place.

The first step to uncovering a possible allergy is to create a baseline of all your current symptoms, from most noticeable to least noticeable, including frequency and detailed descriptions of each—write "nausea with gas" instead of "stomach trouble." Then determine whether you have an allergy by eliminating certain allergy-provoking foods in what is called a General Elimination Diet for three weeks. During this time, avoid:

- *Dairy foods,* including all forms of milk, butter, most margarines, cheese, yogurt, and ice cream. Read food package labels carefully, since many prepared foods are made with dried milk, dried whey, or a milk protein called caseinate. Become a sophisticated reader of labels.

- *Chocolate,* including cocoa products, colas, and some dark rye breads (read the label).

- *Salicylates,* including many preservatives and flavorings; aspirin; toothpaste and chewing gum; almonds; tea; jams and jellies; beer; and a number of fruits and vegetables, including tomatoes, cherries, blackberries, nectarines, and oranges. Because this category is quite large, and because labels do not always warn you about the presence of salicylates, consult an allergist or nutritionist for advice on planning a salicylate-free diet.

Stick to the diet as closely as possible. Afterwards, evaluate the results of only the third week, since the first two weeks are meant to simply cleanse the body. Did your symptoms improve, and if so, by how much compared with your baseline? If your symptoms improved, then you can suspect that a food allergy is causing your problem. If there was no improvement, or only slight improvement, you will have to look in other directions.

Once you have determined that a food allergy is involved, you can pinpoint the offending foods by adding each item, *one at a time*, back to the General Elimination Diet every day for five days, and noting the results. You may find that you cannot eat certain foods at all, but that you can eat limited amounts of others. Be careful with foods such as shellfish, peanuts, or eggs, as these items can provoke particularly strong reactions, especially if you have not eaten them for a while. And always consult your doctor if you are prone to asthma or other potentially life-threatening disorders.

Source: S. Astor. *Hidden Food Allergies*. Garden City Park NY: Avery Publishing Group, 1997.

is the main energy source for the cells that line the large intestine. Butyric acid repairs and regenerates damaged cells.

• *Bentonite clay* absorbs numerous toxins and bacteria. That lowers the amount of toxins present in the intestines, which facilitates healing. (For more information on internal cleansers, see Chapter 11.)

- *Prostaglandin (PG) E2/E1 (Misoprostol)* protects the mucous membrane. Misoprostol reduces the hyperpermeability caused by the taking of indomethacin, a NSAID. Certain substances used by the body to create natural PGE2, such as certain essential fatty acids, also are beneficial.

- *Free radical scavengers* such as the antioxidants vitamin E, beta-carotene, vitamin C, zinc, selenium, and superoxide dismutase fight damage caused by free radicals, which are toxic substances produced when oxygen is processed within the body.

- *Mucus secretion stimulants* encourage the intestinal wall to produce more protective mucus.

- *Digestive enzymes,* such as plant enzymes, hydrochloric acid, pepsin, and pancreatin, help to lessen the amount of toxins present in the intestines by reducing the workload of the intestinal lining, which in turn improves digestion.

- *Probiotic supplements* are by far the most useful means of reducing hyperpermeability. Bacteria in the *Bifidobacteria* and *Lactobacilli* families are very effective in maintaining a healthy gastrointestinal tract (see Chapter 12 and Appendix C).

As we have seen, problems that start in the intestines often do not remain there. Treatment of leaky gut syndrome is important not only for digestive health, but for overall health as well. In the next chapter, we will show you how another intestinal syndrome, the yeast syndrome, can also have wide-ranging effects on health.

CHAPTER 7

How the Yeast Syndrome Affects More Than Just the Digestive System

Growing numbers of doctors in various medical specialties are coming to accept the idea that chronic, generalized, yeast-related illnesses originate in the intestines. These diseases are manifestations of a condition referred to by wholistic physicians as *polysystemic chronic candidiasis* (PSCC), otherwise known as the *yeast syndrome*, and by conventionally trained allergists as *candidiasis hypersensitivity syndrome*.

The yeast syndrome is an infection caused by the fungus family *Candida*, usually involving the species *Candida albicans*, the predominant parasitic yeast present in all of us. This fungus is normally controlled by acids produced by friendly bacteria in the intestinal tract. These bacteria keep the body in a state of balance known as *homeostasis*. If that balance is disrupted, *C. albicans* starts to overgrow and dominate the gut flora, the mix of microbes that normally inhabit the intestines.

Of course, not all doctors agree that the yeast syndrome is a cause of widespread disease, and a number of doctors think it is of little importance. However, more and more physicians are coming to realize that this syndrome is responsible for a number of disorders, both within the intestines and in other areas of the body. In this chapter, we will first explain the various problems associated with the yeast syndrome before turning to the effect candida can have on women's health. We will then discuss ways of treating the yeast syndrome.

HOW THE YEAST SYNDROME AFFECTS THE BODY

Candida can exist in two states: a rounded spore form, which is noninvasive, and a mycelial form, which is invasive. *Mycelia* are the fine, branching threads that make up the growing part of a fungus. In its mycelial form, candida produces long, rootlike structures that can penetrate into the mucous membranes. The amount of mycelia produced is related to the severity of the infection. Yeast can become infectious for a number of reasons, including the use of antibiotics or birth control pills, exposure to molds, poor diet, and stress.

As in the case of bacterial overgrowth, a situation we discussed in Chapter 5, an intestinal yeast infection can produce symptoms in other parts of the body. Such an overgrowth overwhelms the intestinal immune system, thus allowing the yeast and/or its toxins to escape into the bloodstream. The damage done to the mucous membrane in this process also allows undigested food particles to pass through, which causes food allergies (see "Testing for Food Allergies" on page 70 and *Hidden Food Allergies* in Appendix B).[1]

The recognized symptoms and signs of the yeast syndrome include:

- Gastrointestinal problems, including Crohn's disease, irritable bowel syndrome, spastic colon, gastritis, and hemorrhoids (see Chapters 2 and 3)

- Chronic vaginitis (see page 76)
- Brain reactions, including depression, anxiety, paranoia, mania, confusion, forgetfulness, moodiness, and short attention span
- Chronic fatigue
- Fever and flulike feelings
- Frequent urination, burning with urination, and subsequent kidney or bladder infections
- Joint and muscle problems, including weakness, heaviness in the lower limbs, numbness, paralysis or tingling of the extremities, poor coordination, chronic joint pain, joint stiffness, odd swellings, and arthritis
- Itching around the anus, feet, genitals, and other places
- Abdominal bloating, belching, flatulence, and nausea
- Back pain over the kidney area
- Skin problems, including rashes, acne, dryness or oiliness, scaliness or psoriasis, toenail or fingernail fungus, soreness of the digits, and ridges in the nails
- Athlete's foot
- Inflammation along the lymphatic vessels and under the arms
- Upper respiratory problems, including postnasal drip, congestion, and sinusitis
- Carbohydrate cravings
- Generalized swelling and weight gain
- Increased sensitivity to molds and chemicals
- Menstrual problems, including severe abdominal cramping, premenstrual syndrome, and endometriosis

- Allergic reactions, including headaches, earaches, hives, rashes, itching, hay fever, and food cravings or sensitivities

- Sexual dysfunction

- Male reproductive-tract problems, including impotence and prostate trouble

- Lung problems, including persistent coughs and asthma

- Infertility

- Vision problems, including blurring and spots before the eyes

Obviously, you can suffer from one or more of these problems and not have the yeast syndrome. But if you are persistently bothered by a number of the listed disorders and symptoms, we would urge you to seek medical attention. (Children can also suffer from the yeast syndrome—see "Candida and Kids.")

CANDIDA AND WOMEN'S HEALTH

One of the most common candida-related health problems is vaginitis, an inflammation of vulva and vagina that produces discharge, itchiness, redness, and odor. Vaginitis is the result of *vaginosis*, a complex reaction to changes in the types of microbes that inhabit the vagina. *C. albicans* normally inhabits the vagina, but is usually kept in check by good organisms such as those in the *Lactobacilli* family. However, as in the intestines, candida can overgrow in the vagina and produce yeast vaginitis.[2]

While vaginitis can be sexually transmitted, most women who experience recurrent vaginal yeast infections are actually showing signs of a problem that arises from

Candida and Kids

Does your child have:

- Frequent infections, particularly of the ears or tonsils; bronchitis; history of constant diaper rash?

- Continuous nasal congestion or drainage?

- Dark circles under the eyes? Periods of hyperactivity or poor attention span?

These are all signs of the yeast syndrome in children. (In addition, teenage girls, like older women, are prone to yeast vaginitis. Vaginitis is rare in prepubescent girls.) Children are prone to candida problems for the same reasons adults are: too much sugar and too little fiber in the diet, allergy, stress, and overuse of antibiotics. As in the case of adult infection, children with candida respond to proper diet, rest, the use of antifungal treatments as required, and dietary supplementation with probiotics.

Source: J.P. Trowbridge and M. Walker. *Yeast-Related Illnesses.* Greenwich CT: Devin-Adair Publishers, 1987.

yeast overgrowth in the intestines. Because the vagina and the anus are so close together, yeast and bacteria can pass from one to the other. Successful treatment of recurrent candida vaginitis consists of reducing yeast in the large intestine while simultaneously strengthening the body's immune system to resist yeast overgrowth.

Besides *C. albicans*, other members of the *Candida* family that can cause vaginitis include *C. glabrata*, *C. tropicalis*, and *C. torulopsis*. As a general principle, yeasts other than *C. albicans* are more resistant to therapy, requiring longer courses of treatment with higher doses of medication or natural remedies (see page 81). The fungal infection may be accompanied by bacterial infections, or by infection with the parasite *Trichomonas vaginalis.*[3]

Recurrent or chronic candida vaginosis is associated with several contributing factors:

- Heavy colonization of the intestine with candida. Chronic yeast vaginitis can manifest itself as urethral infections and perianal or anal infections. Failure to eliminate candida from the gastrointestinal tract generally results in the return of vaginal yeast infections. Failure to normalize the gut flora with probiotics (see Chapter 12) impedes removal of candida from the digestive system.

- Recurrent antibiotic usage.

- High dietary sugar intake. Women with recurrent yeast vaginitis consume significantly higher amounts of simple carbohydrates.

- The presence of diabetes.

- The use of birth control pills or intrauterine devices (IUDs).

- Vaginal allergy. About 25 percent of all women with recurrent vaginal candiasis have anticandida immune system factors in their vaginal secretions. That results in the release of bodily chemicals which eventually leads to more infection.

- Impaired immune response. A depressed immune response to candida occurs in a small percentage of patients with chronic vaginitis.

Successful treatment of vaginitis consists of:

- Following the yeast-fighting program that is outlined on page 80.

- Taking the appropriate treatment for the entire recommended time, and not just until symptoms disap-
  pear.

- Preventing reinfection from one's sexual partner
  through the use of condoms and by preventing fecal
  contamination of the vagina. Partners of women with
  chronic vaginitis may want to have themselves examined for yeast syndrome.

- Avoiding chemical and mechanical irritants.

- Using preventive measures, such as improved hygiene, undeodorized sanitary napkins instead of tam-
  pons, and natural fiber undergarments.

- Switching to other methods of birth control, if cur-
  rently using birth control pills or an IUD.

- Undergoing tests for diabetes, especially in persistent
  cases.

HOW TO ELIMINATE THE YEAST SYNDROME

For a number of years, the yeast syndrome, except for
yeast vaginitis and oral thrush, was hardly considered
significant by organized medicine. Most physicians treated their patients' candida-related disorders only locally
and seldom systematically, even though yeast overgrowth might affect the entire body. Because the symptoms and signs associated with the yeast syndrome are
sometimes vague and broadly dispersed among a variety of body systems, tissues, and organs, doctors did
not recognize that all the symptoms were from the same
source—an overgrowth of *C. albicans* in the intestines. At
the same time, it is wrong to think you can self-diagnose and self-treat the yeast syndrome. You should
speak to your doctor if you suspect this syndrome is
causing your symptoms. If he or she does not respond

to your concerns, consult an alternative health practitioner. (Also, see *The Yeast Connection*, *The Yeast Syndrome*, and *Yeast-Related Illnesses* in Appendix B.)

The yeast syndrome is similar to the other disorders we have discussed in this book in that treatment requires basic changes in lifestyle, and not just drugs alone. A good yeast-fighting program must include:[4]

- Reducing the amount of simple sugars eaten, including cake, candy, cookies, ice creams, and sugary cereals.

- Decreasing stool transit time by consuming more high-fiber foods (see Chapter 9).

- Avoiding the use of antibiotics, if possible (see "The Dangers of Antibiotics" on page 53).

- Strengthening the natural immune function of the body through proper diet, exercise, and stress reduction, plus the use of immune-enhancing supplements, such as vitamins and minerals

- Use of appropriate medications and natural therapies.

Some substances used to treat candida can selectively interfere with the yeast-to-mycelium transition phase, which makes them more effective against relatively resistant infections.[5] Drug treatment for the yeast syndrome consists of anticandida medicines such as oral nystatin. Other, more powerful, drugs include oral amphotericin B, miconazole, ketoconazole, griseofulvin, candicidin, clotrimazole, and flucytosine. All of these drugs have adverse side effects, with nystatin being by far the least noxious. Some side effects, especially in the case of nystatin, result from the body becoming temporarily overloaded with dead yeast cells and their wastes. This "die-off" effect usually disappears within several days.[6]

A number of natural substances have been found have anticandida properties. They include:

- *Garlic* in all its forms—as raw cloves, oil, tablets, and liquid. Many garlic supplements are available, and all are good for you. One brand, Kyolic aged garlic extract, has been the subject of extensive research, and is effective and odorless (see Appendix C).

- *Caprylic acid*, a fatty acid. It works wonderfully when combined with other substances, such as nystatin. Other fatty acids known as *essential fatty acids* help promote healing.

- *Pau d'arco* (also called lapacho or taheebo), a tea made from the bark of a South American tree. It has antibacterial and blood-cleansing properties, and acts in concert with other substances.

- *B-complex vitamins*, especially biotin and vitamin B_{12}. These vitamins are important to all bodily functions, including digestion, brain function, and infection resistance.

- *Probiotics,* including *Lactobacillus acidophilus, L. fermentum, L. casea, L. salivores, L. brevis, L. plantarum, L. bulgaricus,* and *L. bifidus.*[7] These beneficial bacteria can also be found in fresh, plain yogurt (see Chapters 10 and 12, and Appendix C).

As we have seen in this chapter, an overgrowth of yeast in the intestines may lead to seemingly unrelated disorders throughout the body, especially vaginitis in women. In the next chapter, we will discuss internal parasites, another often unsuspected intestinal problem.

CHAPTER 8

Intestinal Parasites and Chronic Illness

Few people realize the enormous adverse impact on human well-being of parasites and the diarrheal diseases they cause. Worldwide, diarrheal diseases resulting from bacterial and parasitic infection constitute the greatest single cause of disease and death.[1] Numerous medical studies show that up to 99 percent of people living in developing countries suffer from parasitic infections.[2]

In the United States, you may be surprised to learn that diarrheal diseases caused by parasitic infections are the third leading cause of potentially fatal illness. Many Americans assume that intestinal parasites are encountered only in distant parts of the world or in impoverished rural areas.[3] That is simply not true.

In this chapter, we will first discuss a study that shows how anyone can be subject to infection by parasites. We will then explain what parasites are and where they come from, and review the parasites that most commonly infect humans. Finally, we will tell you about the various treatments used to fight parasites.

PARASITES CAN INFECT ANYONE

In the suburban town of Elmhurst, New York, a test sampling of people with digestive complaints showed that fifty-one of sixty-seven patients were found to harbor at least one parasitic organism. The prevalence of these illness-producing creatures, which ranged from microscopic organisms to fifteen-foot-long tapeworms, came as a shock to the populace. Even Elmhurst's doctors—who, like most American doctors, usually receive almost no training in diagnosing and treating parasitic infections—were amazed by the findings.

Until then, the patients' symptoms had been treated empirically. That is, the underlying cause of their diarrhea, abdominal cramping, bloating, gas, and other discomforts were being relieved only with stopgap remedies. Cure was impossible, because the cause of these symptoms—parasites—had not been identified.

"We think of the United States as a highly sanitized country, but that is not necessarily true," said Myron G. Schultz, M.D., Director of the Parasitic Diseases Division of the United States Centers for Disease Control and Prevention in Atlanta, which checked the test results. "Many patients have experienced weeks of delay before the correct diagnosis was made and have been subjected to unnecessary laboratory testing, hospitalization, and even surgery. The large percentage of parasites infecting people . . . means that protozoa and helminths [worms] are causing many diseases that baffle doctors."[4]

The high proportion of parasitic infections discovered in the Elmhurst study may not reflect the actual rate of infection in the general public. But it does reveal that the parasite problem is much more widespread than most health professionals had thought.

WHAT PARASITES ARE AND WHERE THEY COME FROM

Parasites are organisms that live on or within plants or animals of other species, called *hosts*. Parasites obtain nutrients at the host's expense and injure the host through their activities. Parasites differ from *symbionts*, such as the probiotic bacteria discussed in Chapter 12, because symbionts work in concert with their hosts to produce conditions favorable to both creatures. Among the organisms classified as parasites, only some are referred to as *pathogens*, or disease-producing organisms.

Parasitic infections produce a variety of symptoms, including:

- Bloody or foul-smelling stools
- Abdominal pain, cramps, flatulence, and distention
- Anal itching and bleeding
- Diarrhea and/or constipation—diarrhea that lasts more than three days can lead to severe dehydration
- Vomiting and weight loss
- Fever—seek prompt medical attention if fever lasts more than twenty-four hours
- Headaches
- Low back pain
- Skin rash and itching

Parasitic infections are associated with a number of digestive problems, including colitis, Crohn's disease, food allergy, gastritis, inflammatory bowel disease, irritable bowel syndrome, and malabsorption (see Chapters 2 and 3).[5,6] Diagnosis is made through a stool sample.[7]

Parasitic infections are also connected with other disorders, including anorexia, arthritis, autoimmune disease, and chronic fatigue. These diseases may result when the presence of parasites triggers *autoimmune reactivity*, in which the parasite causes tissue destruction. This releases high amounts of substances that, in turn, produce a reaction in which the body attacks itself.[8]

As we mentioned earlier, parasitic infections are common in developing countries. Therefore, worldwide travel by Americans,[9] coupled with increasing immigration, account for a significant number of the parasitic infections seen in the United States. But there are many other sources of infection, including:[10]

- Infected food handlers in places such as restaurants
- Municipal and rural water supplies, especially those contaminated by sewerage
- Day-care centers, where toddlers and young children pass parasites to one another
- Household pets, especially infected cats and dogs
- Foods that generally are eaten raw, such as sushi and steak tartare
- Armed forces personnel returning from overseas
- Sexual contact with multiple partners
- The use of antibiotics and drugs that suppress the immune system
- The spread of AIDS,[11,12] because of the damage AIDS does to the immune system

THE MOST COMMON INTESTINAL PARASITES

Parasites can be classified into two basic groups, protozoa and worms. Some parasites enter the body through the skin or through insect bites; we have limited our discussion to those parasites that enter through the gastrointestinal tract. Various types of bacteria—including the *Salmonella* family, *Listeria monocytogenes*, and *Clostridium botulinum*—also cause food poisoning.

Protozoa are one-celled creatures that can multiply rapidly, taking over the intestines. Some protozoa can hide inside little sacs called *cysts* to protect themselves from the body's defenses, and are often spread in this form. The protozoa that cause disease in humans belong to five groups: amoebae, flagellates, ciliates, coccidia, and microsporidia.[13,14] Most are transmitted through food, water, or other materials contaminated with human or animal stool. Contaminated water supplies are a particular problem, since many protozoan cysts are not killed by usual levels of drinking-water chlorination.

Disease-causing intestinal protozoa include:

- *Blastocystis hominis.* At one laboratory, this organism is found in 20 percent or more of the stool samples received for diagnosis,[15] making it one of the most commonly diagnosed parasites. It is known to be associated with many chronic conditions, including irritable bowel syndrome, chronic fatigue, and arthritic complaints. Often it lodges in the cells of the intestinal lining, making eradication difficult.[16,17]

- *Dientamoeba fragilis.* This is another frequent source of parasitic infections, although it often goes undetected by doctors and laboratory workers alike. It resides in the colon and is transmitted by direct ingestion of the eggs of some worms, especially pinworms (see page 89).[18,19]

- *Entamoeba histolytica.* This organism enters the body in cyst form. Once in the intestines, it assumes the active *trophozoite* form and starts to multiply. From the intestines, it can infect the brain, heart, liver, and lungs, mimicking the symptoms of several serious diseases.

- *Giardia lamblia.* This organism attaches itself via a sucker to the cells lining the duodenum, causing gastroenteritis. When it is swept into the contents of the bowel, *G. lamblia* transforms itself into cysts, which spread from host to host, such as among children in day-care centers.[20] It has a broad geographic distribution and also occurs in waterborne epidemics, which have involved mountain streams, well water, and even some chlorinated water systems. Dr. Leo Galland and Dr. Martin Lee tested patients with inflammatory bowel disease (IBD) and discovered *G. lamblia* in half of them. Treatment for parasites eliminated the IBD symptoms in nine out of ten patients.[21]

- *Endolimax nana.* This is one of the smallest members of the amoeba family. Infection with this organism can provoke an arthritic reaction.

- *Toxoplama gondii.* People usually acquire this parasite from cats, although it can also be found in undercooked meat. It often produces no symptoms at all. Some people, though, develop a mononucleosis-type infection, with fever, headache, and fatigue, and some develop a chronic form of toxoplasmosis, in which hepatitis, swollen lymph glands, and sometimes blindness develop. Pregnant women must make a particular effort to avoid *T. gondii*, especially in the first trimester, as the protozoa can cause blindness, mental retardation, or even death of the unborn child.

- *Cryptosporidium muris* and *parvum.* These are members of another protozoan family that may spread quickly in day-care centers. *Cryptosporidium* usually produces mild infections in healthy patients, but can be life-threatening in patients with faulty immune systems, such as people with AIDS.

- *Entamoeba coli* and *hartmanni*. These organisms are usually harmless. However, virulent strains may cause diarrhea and dysentery.

Intestinal worms are prevalent throughout the world. They are multicellular organisms that produce eggs or larvae, which can be detected in stool specimens. Some of the more commonly occurring worms are:

- *Roundworm (Ascaris lumbricoides).* About 1 billion people worldwide are infected with roundworms, making this organism the most common intestinal parasite.[22] A severe infestation can cause an intestinal blockage. The worms can also travel to the liver, heart, and lungs, where they can cause allergic reactions. Humans may become infected with roundworm species usually found in dogs and cats.

- *Pinworm (Enterobius vermicularis).* Pinworms are the most common intestinal parasites in children, who often put fingers and other objects in their mouths. A pinworm infection causes intense anal itching, its most notable symptom, but can also result in problems with brain function and eyesight.

- *Tapeworm.* Several different species of tapeworm can infect people. All have a head, or *scolex*, that burrows into the intestinal wall, and have segmented bodies. They are the largest intestinal parasites, reaching lengths of several feet. Despite this, some species of tapeworm do not produce many symptoms. However, the pork tapeworm (*Taenia solium*) can cause severe symptoms if larvae invade the heart, eyes, or brain. In the brain, pork tapeworm can result in epileptic-like seizures. The fish tapeworm (*Diphyllobothrium latum*) can absorb all of the host's vitamin B_{12}, producing anemia.

- *Trichinella (Trichuris trichiura)*. While this parasite may be transmitted through stool-contaminated soil, it is also found in pork, and is the reason pork should always be cooked until well done. It is introduced into the body in cyst form. In the intestines, the cysts dissolve, and the worms travel to the muscles, where they produce pain and fever. Other symptoms, including swelling, enlarged lymph glands, and brain inflammations, may result from worms burrowing into various types of tissue.

- *Anisakid worm*. The adult worms live in sea mammals, while the larvae are found in fish such as haddock, herring, cod, red snapper, and Pacific salmon. Eating raw or undercooked fish, such as that used in sushi, can introduce the worms into the intestines, where they can cause inflammation, Crohn's disease, and appendicitis.

- *Strongyloides (Strongyloides stercoralis)*. This parasite enters the body through the skin but travels to the intestines, where it produces nausea, bloating, and diarrhea. It can also travel to the lung, producing respiratory symptoms. Strongyloides can remain in the body for thirty years, and is often found in people with AIDS.

- *Flukes*. There are several species of fluke that are transmitted via infected fish, shellfish, vegetables, and fruit. They are generally found in Asia, with some cases being reported in various parts of the Southern Hemisphere.

ELIMINATING PARASITES FROM THE INTESTINES

Elimination of parasites from the patient's body is the most vital aspect of therapy for parasitic infection. Just relieving the symptoms is not enough. It is important to speak to your doctor or other health care provider when attempting to deal with a parasitic infection, since identification of the specific parasite is important. (See Appendix C and *Guess What Came to Dinner* in Appendix B; for information on how to avoid parasitic infections, see "Cooking to Kill Parasites" on page 92.)

Before the infection itself can be treated, it is important to cleanse the intestinal tract. Enemas can help flush out the lower part of the large intestine. Warm water, garlic juice, vinegar, and blackstrap molasses all make good cleansing enemas. The entire large intestine can be cleansed through colonic irrigation, which must be done by a professional. Various natural laxatives can remove old mucus and encrusted waste material. Psyllium husks, flaxseeds, beet root, bentonite clay, citrus pectin, papaya extract, or agar-agar can be used for this purpose. (For more information on internal cleansing, see Chapter 11.)

It is also important for the patient to eat a proper diet. According to one textbook on parasitology: "The general nutritional status of the host may be of considerable importance both in determining whether or not a particular infection will be accompanied by symptoms, and in influencing their severity if present."[23] Well-cooked poultry and fish, along with well-cooked vegetables, should be the basis of the diet. Soy foodstuffs, including tofu, tempeh, miso, and various soy beverages (see Appendix C), are valuable for their immunity-enhancing effects.

Drugs used in fighting parasitic infections include metronidazole, furazolidone, tinidazole, iodoquinol, paromomycin, and diloxanide furoate. It is important to note, though, that many parasites have developed resistance to these drugs. Also, these drugs may produce serious side effects. Therapy should be stopped promptly if signs of poisoning appear, including heartbeat and

Cooking to Kill Parasites

It seems obvious: The best way to deal with a parasitic infection is to avoid becoming contaminated with parasites, or with the bacterial species that also cause food poisoning, such as *Salmonella*. This task is not as simple as it appears, though. Immune-system stress, increased contact among various parts of the world, and high-speed mechanized meat handling, with its increased risk of bacterial infection, have all led to an increase in the incidence of food poisoning.

The way you select, handle, and cook food can go a long way in protecting you and your family from contamination. The following tips can help you eat safely:

- *Try to buy clean food.* There are no guarantees, since even the most scrupulous of retailers can unwittingly sell contaminated food. That said, you are less likely to get into trouble if you buy your groceries, especially your raw meat and produce, from established dealers and farmstands, not from roadside trucks. Stick with Pacific salmon and red snapper that have been blast-frozen, since these species are known to carry parasites. Also, lean fish, such as cod, flounder, haddock, and sole, are less likely to carry toxic-chemical accumulations when compared with fatty fish, such as bluefish, catfish, or fresh tuna.

- *Use clean water.* Use filtered water at all times. Make sure the filter is fine enough, with a pore size of no more than three microns across, to catch protozoic cysts.

- *Handle all food items as though they are contaminated.* After handling raw meat, fish, or eggs, wash your hands before touching utensils and other foods. Use separate knives and cutting boards for raw meat, raw vegetables, and cooked foods. Marinate raw meat and fish in the refrigerator, and do not baste with the marinade.

- *Disinfect food and vegetables.* Put half a teaspoon of Clorox brand bleach in one gallon of filtered water. Use this solution to disinfect cutting boards and cooking utensils, and to soak raw meat and produce. Soaking times range from fifteen minutes for leafy vegetables and thin-skinned fruits; to twenty minutes for poultry, fish, meat, and eggs; to thirty minutes for root vegetables and thick-skinned fruits. Afterwards, rinse all food items by soaking them in plain filtered water for ten minutes. Dry foods thoroughly before using or storing.

- *Avoid certain dishes.* Unless you really know what you are doing, do not attempt to make sushi, steak tartare, and other raw fish- or meat-based foods at home. Cook your eggs until they are no longer runny, and stay away from recipes that call for raw eggs, such as homemade mayonnaise. Do not eat raw shellfish.

- *Cook meat thoroughly.* Cook meat and poultry until it is no longer pink inside, and fish until it is flaky and white. Better yet, use a meat thermometer to ensure that fish reaches an internal temperature of at least 140°F; beef, 160°F; lamb, veal, and pork, 170°F; and poultry, 180°F.

- *Do not sample suspect foods.* Do not taste fish or meat dishes before they are done, and do not eat egg-based batter.

- *Police your kitchen.* Keep your knives and cutting boards scrupulously clean with Clorox solution, and throw away boards that are badly pitted and gouged. Microwave your sponges on high for thirty to sixty seconds, or run them (and your dishrags) through the dishwasher. Use paper towels for spills.

Sources: A.L. Gittleman. *Guess What Came to Dinner.* Garden City Park NY: Avery Publishing Group, 1993; C.S. DeWaal. Clean fish, dirty fish. *Nutrition Action Healthletter* 21(9):8, 1994; Kitchen hygiene. *Nutrition Action Healthletter* 22(3):6, 1995; The safe food kitchen. *Nutrition Action Healthletter* 23(6):8, 1996.

blood-pressure irregularities, muscular weakness, intestinal symptoms, and skin lesions.

Antiparasitic herbs have been used since long before drugs were ever invented. Some of the most potent herbs are black walnut bark, butternut root bark, artemesia, garlic, pinkroot, goldenseal, wormwood, sage, clove, tansy, fennel, thyme, cranberry powder, and male fern. These herbs have been formulated into various commercial formulas; see Appendix C for more information, or consult an herbalist.

Homeopathic therapies are particularly effective against worms. Homeopathy is based on the idea that "like cures like," and uses extremely small dosages of substances that, in larger amounts, can induce symptoms. See a homeopathic doctor if you wish to explore this option.

Once the intestines are cleared of parasites, it is important to restock the system with friendly bacteria. This is best done through the consumption of plain, fresh yogurt, and through supplementation with probiotics (see Chapters 10 and 12, and Appendix C).

Good food and travel are two of life's pleasures, and we would not discourage you from enjoying either of them. It is important to remember, though, that parasitic infections are more common than you think. Do not dismiss signs of infection as "just a stomachache" or "a touch of the flu."

Now that we have looked at the problem of indigestion, it is time to look at the solution. In the next chapter, we will discuss the Mediterranean diet, and how it can help keep your gastrointestinal tract—and the rest of your body—healthy.

PART TWO

Indigestion Solutions

The supermarket and pharmacy shelves are full of heartburn and other indigestion remedies, all promising faster, more effective relief. But as we have seen, the relief these pills and potions provide is temporary, at best. They may address the symptoms of indigestion, but do not deal with its root causes—the gastrointestinal disorders that we discussed in Part One.

In this part, we will give you ways to find lasting relief from both the symptoms *and* the causes of indigestion. Because proper diet is such a fundamental part of digestive health, we will first explain how the Mediterranean diet can give you the sound nutrition you need. We will then discuss the benefits of yogurt, and of fiber and other intestinal cleansers. Finally, we will show you how the use of probiotics can banish indigestion for good.

CHAPTER 9

Achieving Digestive Health Through Proper Diet

The first part of the indigestion solution involves eating a proper diet. Remember, the modern glut of fat, sugar, and salt is simply not normal when seen in the light of human history. The bodies of our prehistoric ancestors became adapted to scarcity, especially a scarcity of calories. All but the wealthiest of people lived with such scarcity, or the threat of it, throughout the ages until the Industrial Revolution brought about drastic alterations in the production, processing, and distribution of food. The available amounts of both calories and salt have increased greatly, but the human body has changed very little since prehistoric times.[1,2] As a result, people of the past actually experienced far less degenerative disease—heart disease and stroke, cancer, and the digestive disorders discussed in Part One—than people living in today's industrialized countries.[3]

Eating a proper diet means consuming more natural foods, many of them raw if possible, along with more vitamins and minerals, and reduced amounts of animal products. It also means eating fewer highly refined foods, with a corresponding decrease in intakes of fat, salt, and preservatives. These principles form the basis of the modified Mediterranean diet that we recommend. Osteopathic physician and author Cass Igram says, "If you follow the standard American diet, your eating habits are creating severe nutritional deficiencies," generally in the B-complex vitamins, minerals, and essential fatty acids (see page 104).[4]

In this chapter, we will first provide a good digestive-health diet, and then show you how to modify this diet to meet the nutritional challenges posed by different gastrointestinal disorders.

EATING RIGHT FOR GOOD HEALTH

The following diet is based on the popular Mediterranean diet, which in turn is based in large part on the benefits of olive oil.

A Modified Mediterranean Diet

Inasmuch as there are more than a dozen Mediterranean nations with varied cultures, traditions, and dietary habits, the Mediterranean diet is not a uniform nutritional model. However, the diets of all these countries have some things in common, items that include:[5]

- Low amounts of saturated fat
- High amounts of monounsaturated fat, thanks to the extensive use of olive oil
- Moderate amounts of animal protein
- High amounts of carbohydrates
- High amounts of vegetables and leguminous fiber

Of all the traditional Mediterranean diets, the healthiest is Greek cuisine.[6] Greeks who follow a traditional diet eat more fish, legumes, vegetables, fruits, and cereal grains than do Americans. They drink more wine, and eat less meat and fewer eggs. They have a life expectancy at age forty-five that is higher than that of people living in the United States, and fewer cases of coronary heart disease and cancer.

The Greek diet is considered optimal, although other factors besides diet, such as genetics, environmental pollutants, and amounts of sunlight, also differ between the United States and Greece. But diet is the most important factor in accounting for the differences in health statistics between the two countries. In fact, all the peoples living along the Mediterranean coast are healthier than Americans, because the former eat fewer commercially prepared and processed foods, almost no fast foods, and near-zero amounts of junk foods. Unfortunately, adoption of a modern diet and lifestyle has led to increases in obesity, diabetes, and cardiovascular diseases among these Mediterranean populations.

Our modified Mediterranean diet consists of:[7]

- *Whole-grain breads, pastas, and cereals.* Whole grains are much more nutritious than their refined counterparts, with more fiber, vitamins, minerals, and essential fatty acids. Good grains include whole wheat, oats, whole grain cornmeal, buckwheat, brown rice, and barley.

- *Raw or lightly steamed vegetables and sprouts, plus raw fruit.* Fruits and vegetables contain not only fiber, vitamins, and minerals, but also generous amounts of phytochemicals, substances that benefit health. Cooking destroys many of these nutrients. Eat the nutrient-rich skins of fruits such as apples and pears, but be sure to wash your produce well in order to avoid pesticide residues and parasitic infections (Chapter 8).

- *Cooked beans, lentils, and peas, and raw, unsalted nuts and seeds.* Beans, lentils, and peas are all members of the legume family, which is a rich source of protein, potassium, and fiber. One bean, the soybean, is the basis of the traditional Asian foods tofu and miso, and of the "fake meats" widely available in American supermarkets. Nuts and seeds are also rich sources of nutrients—just be aware that they are high in calories.

- *Fresh meat, fish, and poultry in small amounts to complement the vegetables, grains, and legumes.* Meat, a fine source of protein, is not evil. But it does contain high amounts of cholesterol and saturated fat, and modern methods of production use antibiotics in the animals' feed, which poses a threat to human health (see page 53). Therefore, eat only lean cuts of organically grown meat and poultry. On the other hand, fatty fish, especially cold-water fish, such as salmon, is an excellent source of essential fatty acids.

- *Nonhomogenized dairy products in limited amounts, particularly cultured products such as yogurt.* Yogurt is an important part of Mediterranean cooking, and with good reason: It is nutritious, highly digestible, and full of probiotic bacteria (see Chapter 10). Reduce the use of cow's milk, which can lead to mucus formation in some people. Use limited amounts of cheese in cooking every once in a while. Cheese is a Mediterranean staple, but remember that cheeses such as Greek feta are part of a cuisine that is much lower in fat overall than the standard American diet.

- *Olive oil instead of other oils and cooking fats.* See page 101.

- *Savory flavors to substitute for salt.* Herbs, garlic, and lemon juice provide valuable nutrients, and make your food tasty enough so that you won't reach for the salt shaker.

- *Clean water, green tea, and, for those who drink alcohol, red wine.* Make sure the water you drink is bottled or filtered. Use some of it to make green tea, which provides vitamins, minerals, and amino acids; promotes the growth of probiotic bacteria; protects the gastrointestinal tract against cancer-causing agents; and may help prevent ulcers[8] (see *The Green Tea Book* in Appendix B). If you like a drop of the grape now and then, drink moderate amounts of red wine. It contains substances called oligomeric proanthocyamidins (OPCs), powerful antioxidants that support the work of vitamin C in the body.

Do not consume highly processed foods containing artificial flavorings and preservatives. These foods are totally devoid of nutrients, and actually harm health. Eat sweets rarely, and save soft drinks and hard liquor for special occasions. We do realize that most people are not able to eat properly all the time, and that indigestion can result. If this happens to you, see "Natural Stomach Soothers" on page 102.

The Nutritional Value of Olive Oil

The diets of the United States and Greece differ in the type of cooking oil used. The backbone of the Greek diet is olive oil, and Greece, along with Italy, Spain, Turkey, Morocco, and Portugal, is a major producer of olive oil.

While growing numbers of Americans are now using olive oil, the American diet generally contains a lot of artery-clogging saturated fat from meat and butter. It also contains *polyunsaturated fats* from corn, sunflower, and safflower oils. These oils, once thought of as a

Natural Stomach Soothers

Even if you try to be careful about what you eat, the temptations of modern life do not always encourage a healthy diet: fast food at an airport, chips and dip at a party, cake at a wedding, too much food at any time. When you do overindulge, there are gentle, natural ways of calming your stomach:

- *Papaya* contains enzymes that help speed digestion, and also provides vitamins C and E. The tablets are easy to use.

- *Anise seeds* can be chewed to relieve indigestion. They are also effective against respiratory infections.

- *Ginger* is a powerful stomach soother that reduces spasms and cramps—just don't take too much, or it can cause even more stomach distress. If the fresh root is not available, make a tea of the dried powder. Some people use candied ginger to prevent seasickness.

- *Fennel* relieves abdominal pain and dispels gas, and is especially good for relieving an acid stomach. It also promotes liver, spleen, and kidney function.

- *Peppermint*, a popular flavoring agent, can ease distress in all parts of the gastrointestinal tract. It also stimulates the appetite.

- *Aloe vera* soothes the stomach and provides a gentle laxative effect. When used externally, it is an excellent burn and wound healer.

- *Catnip* aids digestion. Despite its stimulating effect on cats, this herb tends to relieve stress and promote sleep in humans.

- *Fenugreek* lubricates the intestines and acts as a laxative. It also contains vitamins A, B, and D.

● *Charcoal tablets,* available in health food stores, can absorb gas and toxins from the intestines. They can also absorb medications and nutrients, so take them separately, and do not use them for long periods of time.

Hard-to-digest sugars are responsible for the flatulence and bloating that can occur after you eat legumes and other gas-producing vegetables. In this case, try Beano, an over-the-counter digestive aid that breaks down the offending sugars, and thus reduces gas production. If you make beans a regular part of your diet, your system will eventually adjust to them and produce less gas.

heart-disease solution, have been found to promote the development of inflammatory conditions, blood clots, and high blood pressure, especially when used to excess. The American diet also contains artificially created fats called *trans-fatty acids,* which are harmful to health. Present in refined nut butters, margarine, salad dressings, shortenings, and frying oils, trans-fatty acids make up between 5 and 15 percent of the total calories available to North Americans.[9]

Olive oil is a *monosaturated fat,* like that found in avocados, peanuts, almonds, and cashews, and as such, has no known harmful effects. Because the Mediterranean diet relies so heavily on olive oil, it tends to crowd out the kinds of unhealthy fats found in the American diet. Olive oil has been found to contain vitamin E and other antioxidants.[10] This allows it to reduce the oxidation of low-density lipoproteins (LDL), the "bad cholesterol" that, when oxidized, builds up within arteries.[11] It has also been found to reduce levels of LDL and raise levels of high-density lipoproteins (HDL), the "good cholesterol" that helps clear fats out of the bloodstream.[12] Olive oil also contains a chemical called squalene, which helps to oxygenate tissues.

Olive oil also contains *essential fatty acids* (EFA), or fats that your body needs but cannot create itself. There are two main types of EFAs: omega-3 and omega-6. While both are necessary to good health, the American diet tends to supply too much omega-6 and too little omega-3. Olive oil contains about 11 percent omega-6 and 0.8 percent omega-3. Therefore, we recommend that you balance out the omega-6 present in olive oil by taking some flaxseeds or a little flaxseed oil every day, since flaxseed is high in omega-3 (see *Omega 3 Oils* in Appendix B).

Keep in mind that like any oil, olive oil is high in calories. Be sure to balance your calorie intake with your energy expenditure, especially if you are trying to lose weight.

TAILORING THE DIET TO MEET YOUR NEEDS

The modified Mediterranean diet provides a sound basis for optimal digestive health. There are times, though, when you will need to tailor this diet to the needs created by a preexisting gastrointestinal disorder. If you have any of the following disorders, be sure to discuss matters of diet with your doctor.

Tailoring the Diet if You Have Ulcers

As we saw in Chapter 4, doctors now know that ulcers are caused by infection with the *Helicobacter pylori* bacterium, and the traditional bland diet is of little use in curing the infection itself. However, it is still important for someone with ulcers to eat a suitable diet. Therefore, we recommend that until your ulcers heal, you should follow a fairly bland diet eaten in frequent, small

meals. You should consume moderate amounts of protein and plenty of dark green vegetables. Also drink
plenty of green juices, including barley, alfalfa, wheat,
and freshly made cabbage, as these juices promote healing. Fibrous vegetables, such as broccoli and carrots,
should be well steamed. Avoid acidic foods, such as citrus foods and vinegar, along with coffee, black tea, and
alcohol. Soured milk products, such as yogurt, are good,
but avoid regular milk. Despite the immediate relief
milk provides, it stimulates even more acid production,
so try almond or soy milk instead. Supplement your
diet with probiotics (see Chapter 12).

Tailoring the Diet if You Have Constipation

Since the most common cause of constipation is a low-
fiber diet, it stands to reason that a high-fiber diet is
part of the treatment (see Chapter 11). Raw fruits,
prunes and figs, raw leafy green vegetables, brown rice,
asparagus, beans, cabbage, peas, sweet potatoes, and
whole-wheat cereals are just some of the foods that provide healthy amounts of fiber. Take psyllium seeds and
other plant seeds, such as sunflower, pumpkin, and
sesame. Use bran supplements, but do not take large
amounts of bran, which can irritate the intestinal lining.
Remember that as your fiber consumption goes up, so
should your water consumption. Avoid fatty or spicy
foods and dairy products (except for yogurt), as these
foods may encourage mucus production.

Tailoring the Diet if You Have
the Yeast Syndrome

The yeast syndrome occurs when there is an overgrowth
of *Candida albicans*, a harmful yeast that is normally kept
in check by the body's probiotic bacteria (see Chapter

7). If you are troubled by this syndrome, we recommend the meat, eggs, vegetables, yogurt (MEVY) diet, a four-phase diet that controls *C. albicans*. In phase one, which lasts three weeks, the diet is strictly limited, and includes no yeast-based foods or foods that can stimulate yeast growth, such as mushrooms, fruits, and processed foods. Vegetables, fish, millet, and brown rice are all allowed. In phase two, which may last up to three months, some dairy foods are added back to the diet. In phase three, which may last up to a year, sugary natural foods, such as pears, apples, and bananas, are added back to the diet. In phase four, which lasts indefinitely, moderate amounts of yeast-containing and high-carbohydrate foods are included in the diet. (For more information on the complete MEVY diet, see *The Yeast Syndrome* in Appendix B.) Both yogurt and distilled water are recommended throughout the diet, along with fiber and probiotic supplements (see Chapters 11 and 12).

Tailoring the Diet if You Have a Malabsorption or Intolerance Disorder

These disorders include conditions under which the body cannot adequately absorb nutrients from the intestines (see Chapter 2). If you have problems with food absorption or intolerance, we recommend that you avoid all processed and fried foods, alcohol, chocolate, black tea, coffee, and carbonated beverages, especially cola products. Avoid citrus fruits, and peel all other fruits. Do eat a lot of fresh papaya and pineapple, which contain digestive enzymes, and chew four to six papaya tablets after meals. Avoid shellfish, but do eat fin fish several times a week. Greatly reduce your meat consumption, which should be limited to *lean* ham, lamb, veal, or white-meat chicken. Use fats and oils very sparingly. Also use milk sparingly, and limit your dairy consumption to Lactaid or nonfat milk, yogurt, and small amounts of cheese. Avoid hard-fiber wheat cereals and white rice. If you experience no symptoms after thirty days, you can try adding some of the avoided foods back to your diet, but only one at a time and in small amounts.

Tailoring the Diet if You Have a Diarrheal Disorder or Parasitic Infection

In Chapter 2, we saw how diarrhea can be caused by a number of things, including stress, spoiled food, and parasitic infections (see Chapter 8). An old folk remedy for diarrhea calls for an apple, a banana, and cottage cheese to be eaten together. Soft soluble-fiber foods, such as creamy oatmeal, Cream of Wheat, mashed potatoes, and well-cooked brown rice, are also good. Avoid dairy products, but do maintain a good fluid intake. Drink plenty of water, including rice water, which is made by boiling a half-cup of brown rice in three cups of water for forty-five minutes. Rice water helps form stool. Also take hot carob-powder drink, which helps halt diarrhea.

Tailoring the Diet if You Have an Inflammatory Bowel or Irritable Bowel Syndrome

The term "inflammatory bowel disease" covers Crohn's disease, which affects the small intestine, and ulcerative colitis, which affects the large intestine. Irritable bowel syndrome (IBS) is marked by abdominal pain with diarrhea and constipation (see Chapter 2). If you have one of these conditions, we recommend that you avoid processed, fatty, and spicy foods, along with coffee, black tea, alcohol, carbonated beverages, meat, and dairy products. You should also avoid high-fiber cereals, such as All-Bran, and the fibrous parts of fruits, such as apple and pear skins. Eat baked or well-steamed nonacidic vegetables, such as asparagus, broccoli, Brussels sprouts, cabbage, carrots, celery, garlic, kale, spinach, and turnips. Eat broiled or baked fin fish. Add papaya to your diet, both fresh and in tablet form. Use psyllium powder to remove toxins from the intestinal wall, and probiotic supplements to support a healthy gut flora (see Chapter 12). Drink plenty of liquids, including herbal teas and fresh juices—cabbage juice is especially good. During acute attacks, try limiting your diet to organic baby foods.

Tailoring the Diet if You Have a Diverticular Disease

Diverticular diseases include diverticulosis, or the development of little sacs called diverticula in the walls of the large intestine, and diverticulitis, which occurs when these sacs become inflamed (see Chapter 2). If you have one of these conditions, it is important not to irritate the sacs. Therefore, we recommend that you avoid processed, fatty, and spicy foods, along with alcohol, chocolate, coffee, black tea, dairy products, orange and tomato juices, and peppermint and spearmint. Also avoid grains and seeds, except for well-cooked brown rice, as these can become trapped in the sacs. Do consume at least thirty grams of fiber a day, along with plenty of water. Do not use bran as your only source of supplemental fiber, as too much bran can promote gas formation. Eat a high-protein diet that includes plenty of fish, leafy green vegetables, and garlic. During an acute attack, reduce your fiber intake, and put all vegetables and fruits through a blender. An alternative is eat organic baby food until healing takes place.

Tailoring the Diet if You Have Hemorrhoids or Other Anal Disorders

Hemorrhoids, a condition in which veins in the anal area become enlarged and irritated, is one of a number of anal disorders (see Chapter 3). At the first sign of a hemorrhoid attack, it may be helpful to eat a low-fiber, low-residue diet until the pain and itching subside. Between attacks, switch to a high-fiber diet that includes fresh fruit and vegetables, whole-grain cereals, and plenty of water. Spicy foods, peppers, and garlic are all known to irritate hemorrhoids, although peeled garlic cloves, used three times a week, are good suppositories. Blackstrap molasses, alfalfa, and leafy green vegetables are all good sources of vitamin K, which can help heal bleeding hemorrhoids.

We think the modified Mediterranean diet presented in this chapter can lessen your chances of experiencing heartburn and indigestion, especially if you suffer from these problems on a chronic basis. In the next chapter, we will take a closer look at one of the diet's featured items—yogurt.

CHAPTER 10

The Many Benefits of Yogurt

As we saw in Chapter 1, Americans spend billions of dollars each year on antacids, and the temporary relief provided by these drugs is sometimes harmful in the long run. The money spent in the supermarket's pharmacy department would be better spent in the dairy aisle—on smooth, soothing yogurt.

The consumption of yogurt is an ancient practice mentioned in the Bible, and yogurt is featured in national cuisines from Tunisia to India. Its recent reputation as a health food has increased sales: More than 30 percent of the world's population eats yogurt regularly,[1] including a significant number of Americans.

In this chapter, we will describe the many benefits of yogurt, including its effects on the digestive system, before telling you how to ensure that your yogurt is as healthful as possible.

YOGURT: HEARTBURN RELIEF AND MUCH MORE

Fermented milk products, such as yogurt, have been the basis for nutrition and health among cultures ranging across Asia, Africa, Europe, South America, and Australia. Yogurt is made by using certain strains of bacteria, mostly from the *Lactobacillus* family, to thicken and curdle milk. This process gives yogurt not only its characteristic sour taste, but also its health-giving properties.

Yogurt has long been eaten to promote digestive health. The bacteria in yogurt break down protein, making it easier for the resulting amino acids to be absorbed in the digestive tract. These bacteria also predigest lactose, the sugar found in milk, by producing the enzyme lactase. This allows people who suffer from lactose intolerance, and thus are unable to consume milk products, to eat yogurt.

Yogurt's greatest gastrointestinal benefit, however, is its ability to reduce the amount of disease-causing microbes, and the toxins they produce, within the intestines. As we saw in Chapter 5, a state of imbalance, or dysbiosis, develops when bad bacteria in the intestines start to overwhelm the good bacteria. This dysbiosis can lead to disorders in both the digestive tract itself and the body at large, including life-threatening illnesses such as bowel cancer. The bacteria in yogurt, being probiotic (see Chapter 12), can help restore the intestines to a state of health.

Lactobacillus acidophilus, a primary strain of yogurt-making bacteria, suppresses the growth of *Escherichia coli* and *Salmonella typhimurim*, two foodborne pathogens.[2] In fact, a number of the probiotic bacteria found in yogurt produce a range of antibiotic substances (see Table 9.1). Synthetic antibiotics, on the other hand, promote dysbiosis by killing off the friendly intestinal microbes. That is why acidophilus yogurt or capsules is often recommended to people who must take synthetic antibiotics. Acidophilus can also be used to both prevent and treat traveler's diarrhea.[3]

Table 9.1.
Antibiotic Compounds Produced by Probiotic Bacteria

Probiotic Species	Antibiotic Compound
L. acidophilus	Acidolin, Acidophilin, Lactocidin, Bacteriocin Protein
L. brevis	Lactobacillin, Lactobrevin
L. bulgaricus	Bulgarican
L. planarum	Lactolin

In addition to aiding digestion, yogurt provides a number of other health benefits:

- Yogurt contains healthy amounts of several important nutrients, including the B vitamins, especially folic acid, and calcium, a third more than milk cup for cup. In addition, commercially produced yogurt is often thickened with milk solids, and thus contains more protein than plain milk.

- Experiments have shown that milk cultured with friendly bacteria significantly reduces the blood cholesterol level in rats. Yogurt may also have the same effect in humans, although some strains of bacteria are more effective than others in this regard.[4] It has been noted that African Masai warriors, who drink about two quarts of fermented milk a day, have low levels of cholesterol in their bloodstreams.[5]

- One strain of *L. acidophilus*, DDS1, has been shown to inhibit the growth of certain cancer cells, and European studies have found a reduced incidence of breast cancer among people who eat large amounts of yogurt and other fermented milks.[6] Yogurt has several anticancer properties. It can prevent potentially carcinogenic substances, including bile salts, in the intestines from actually becoming carcinogenic, and can keep such harmful substances from being absorbed by the body. Yogurt can also reduce the level of unhealthy enzymes in the stool. In one study, cancer-promoting stool bacteria were three times less active in patients fed milk that contained *L. acidophilus* every day for four weeks when compared with that found in patients fed regular milk.[7]

- Yogurt has been shown to boost the body's ability to fight invaders by increasing the amount of such immune-system components as natural killer cells, macrophages, interferon, and antibodies.[8,9] One study showed that people who ate active-culture yogurt on a regular basis saw their nasal allergy symptoms decrease when compared with people who ate heat-treated yogurt.[10]

- The bacteria in yogurt reduce the overgrowth of the fungus *Candida albicans*, which causes the yeast syndrome (see Chapter 7). "The acidophilus bacteria are natural enemies of yeast," according to Eileen Hilton, M.D., an infectious disease specialist at Long Island Jewish Medical Center in New York. "We think that they colonize . . . the gastrointestinal tract, [and] then migrate to the vagina, where they take up residence and remain to help fight off yeast infections."[11] In a study conducted by Dr. Hilton, thirteen women experienced one-third fewer vaginal yeast infections after they started eating one cup of acidophilus yogurt daily when compared with the experience of these same women over the previous six months.[12]

- There is also evidence that the consumption of yogurt is a basic part of a longevity lifestyle. Russian bacteriologist Elie Metchnikoff, whom we first met in Chapter 5, was convinced that the destructive intestinal microbes to which we are all are exposed each day could be counteracted by the advantageous microbes found in yogurt, which he said "lessened the negative consequences of intestinal putrefaction."[13] He fed a microbe he developed called *Lactobacillus bulgaris* to mice, which caused them to live longer and give birth to more offspring. And yogurt is a dietary staple among the Vilcabambans of Ecuador, people who are known for living well past the century mark.[14,15]

HOW TO ENSURE THAT YOUR YOGURT IS ACTIVE

Yogurt can be made from a great variety of milk products: skim milk, buttermilk, sour cream, sheep's milk, goat's milk. The most important factor is not the sort of milk you start with, but the kind of bacteria, or *starter*, used to culture that milk. Some strains of bacteria are more effective than others in promoting health, and no bacteria is useful unless it is properly active. This is important whether you buy your yogurt or make it yourself.

Buying High-Quality Yogurt

Manufactured yogurt is available in three basic varieties: standard, low-fat, and nonfat. The milk used to make yogurt may be *homogenized*, or made uniform in consistency, and must be *pasteurized*, or heated to kill harmful bacteria, before the starter is added. The starter, being the most important ingredient, is judged on a number of performance factors, such as rapid acid development and survivability of the yogurt-forming bacteria during storage.[16]

Whether the yogurt you buy is healthful or not depends on two factors: the bacteria used to make it and whether those bacteria are alive at the time of purchase. *L. acidophilus*, the hardiest strain, is not used as often by American manufacturers as other strains because it creates a yogurt with too much tang for the United States market. Also, manufacturers sometimes heat-treat yogurt to extend its shelf life. However, this kills off the bacteria altogether, and greatly reduces the yogurt's health benefits.

To ensure that you are getting the best-quality yogurt, become an informed consumer. Carefully check the labels of the different yogurts, looking for products that have not been heat-treated and that do contain at least some *L. acidophilus*. If the product passes these checks, make sure it has enough bacteria per serving—at least 107 organisms per gram, according to criteria established by the National Yogurt Association.[17] If you do not find this information on the label, do not hesitate to contact the manufacturer (see Appendix C for some recommended brands). We would also recommend that you purchase plain yogurt and add your own flavorings, using a minimum of sweetener. Buying yogurt that is full of sugar defeats the purpose of eating yogurt in the first place.

Making High-Quality Yogurt

Depending on which starter is used, homemade yogurt is known to be a rich source of not only *L. acidophilus* but also of *L. bulgaricus* and *Streptococcus thermophilus*, two temporary, or transient, bacteria that perform a number of useful roles within the intestines (see Chapter 12). It is important to keep in mind, though, that each person harbors a slightly different mix of bacteria.[18]

As in commercial manufacture, the starter is the most crucial component in the production of homemade yogurt. Usually, you can acquire the appropriate yogurt starter

Shake Your Yogurt

One of the easiest and most delicious ways to enjoy yogurt is in a cool, refreshing blender drink. The following are just a few ideas. Let your imagination be your guide!

Carrot Shake

1 cup carrot juice
1 cup vanilla-flavored low-fat yogurt
1 medium-sized ripe banana, sliced
1 teaspoon vanilla extract
2 ice cubes

Put all the ingredients in a blender, and blend until smooth. If you want to cut calories, use nonfat yogurt and only half a banana.

Mid-Morning Pickup

½ cup prune juice
½ cup apple juice
2 tablespoons creamy peanut butter
½ cup plain low-fat yogurt

Put all the ingredients into a blender, and blend until smooth. To cut the calories, use nonfat yogurt and reduced-fat peanut butter.

Peach Smoothie

½ cup light tofu, drained
1 cup peach-flavored low-fat yogurt
½ cup peach slices, canned or fresh
1 or 2 ice cubes

Put all the ingredients into a blender, and blend until smooth. To cut the calories, use nonfat yogurt and fresh peach slices.

Source: McMillan L., Jarvie J., and Brauer J. *Positive Cooking.* Garden City Park NY: Avery Publishing Group, 1997, pp. 114, 118, and 120.

from a health food store or a manufacturer who specializes in culturing the appropriate organisms. If you are using a yogurt maker, be sure to first read the directions carefully.

An alternative way to create homemade yogurt starter is to break open six acidophilus capsules—Kyo-Dophilus is a good brand—and add the contents to regular milk, skim milk, sweet cream, buttermilk, sour cream, or cottage cheese.

Once you start making your own yogurt, you will find a number of uses for it besides breakfast and snacks. Depending on the milk it's made from, yogurt is an excellent low-fat alternative to sour cream in dips, dressings, and shakes (see "Shake Your Yogurt" on page 117). It also works well in a variety of baked goods, casseroles, and sauces. Just keep in mind that whenever you heat yogurt, you will kill or weaken the bacteria it contains. So go ahead and create in the kitchen, but make sure you still eat uncooked yogurt in some form every day.

Yogurt has been a health food for at least 4,000 years, and is a delicious way of getting the probiotic bacteria you need for a healthy digestive system. In Chapter 12, we will explain probiotics in greater detail. But first, in the next chapter, we will discuss internal cleansers, including fiber.

CHAPTER 11

Internal Cleansing for Intestinal Health

A healthy intestinal tract is an active tract, one in which food moves along quickly. When waste moves too slowly through the system, it tends to stagnate and create toxins. These toxins, in turn, are responsible for many of the disorders we discussed in Part One. The digestive tract operates properly when there is adequate bulk in the system, since the muscles in the intestinal wall, like muscles elsewhere, need resistance to work against. Fiber, found in the indigestible parts of your food, provides this bulk, and thus promotes intestinal health. It and other natural-laxative substances can return a dysfunctional bowel to normal.

As we have seen, intestinal health also requires the presence of probiotic bacteria to keep disease-promoting microbes at bay (see Chapter 12). Whey preparations feed these good bacteria, as does a special form of carbohydrate called FOS. In this chapter, we will explain how to use a variety of substances to keep your intestinal tract healthy.

NORMALIZING INTESTINAL FUNCTION WITH FIBER AND OTHER SUBSTANCES

The modern diet contains woefully inadequate amounts of fiber, much less than the recommended 25 to 40 grams a day. This may very well explain why so many people are troubled by constipation. Adequate amounts of *insoluble* fiber absorb excess water and toxic wastes, and create soft stools that are easy to pass. This reduces the amount of time that wastes remain in the intestines, which in turn eases both bowel and anal disorders. Some researchers also believe that the bulkier stools created by insoluble fiber reduces the pressure on the large intestine, and thus reduces the risk of diverticulosis.[1]

Adequate amounts of *soluble* fiber soak up bile acids, which are made of cholesterol, in the intestines. This forces the body to pull more cholesterol out of the bloodstream for bile production, and thus reduces blood cholesterol levels—depending on how much fiber you eat.[2] High cholesterol levels are associated with heart disease, and one study did show a correlation between a high fiber intake and a lower risk of heart attack.[3] Soluble fiber also helps to stabilize blood-sugar levels. This is an important consideration for older people, as blood-sugar levels tend to increase with age.

Although a number of excellent fiber supplements are available (see Appendix C), you should obtain most of your daily fiber from your diet. The following foods contain healthy amounts of fiber:

• Bran cereals, oatmeal, brown rice, buckwheat, millet, bulgur wheat, and whole-grain breads and pastas

• Fresh fruits and vegetables, especially apples, peas, baked potatoes with skins left on (both white and sweet), pears, Brussels sprouts, broccoli, oranges, bananas, cabbage, and carrots

- Pulses, such as black or pinto beans, lentils, and chickpeas

- Preservative-free dried fruit, such as figs, apricots, prunes, and dates, all of which should be soaked in water before eating

- Seeds, such as sesame, flax, sunflower, pumpkin, fenugreek, and fennel

We recommend that you obtain the majority of your dietary fiber from fresh fruits and vegetables, and from pulses such as beans. These foods are all low in fat—although, in the case of beans, not low in calories—and full of important nutrients. Add flaxseeds to salads and yogurt, as they contain both fiber and essential fatty acids. Use cold-pressed oils, such as olive, safflower, walnut, and sesame, for their laxative effect. If you do consume supplemental bran, use the loose bran, since the bran tablets may be eliminated before they completely break down. (For a good way to combine the benefits of bran and yogurt, see "An Appetizer for Health" on page 122. For more information on diet in general, see Chapter 9.)

Make purified water your principal daily beverage, and generally avoid tea (except for green tea—see page 101), coffee, soda water, or alcohol (except for red wine). Try to drink one six-ounce glass of water just before each meal, plus three glasses between meals. Water will give fiber the bulk it needs to be an effective cleanser and constipation remedy.

Adding too much fiber to your diet at one time can cause gas and loose stools, particularly if you have been eating a low-fiber diet. Add fiber gradually, and make sure to drink enough fluid. See your doctor before increasing your fiber intake if you have a preexisting intestinal disorder.

An Appetizer for Health

Eat this yogurt-fiber appetizer before each meal. It also makes a filling snack.

1 tablespoon miller's bran or oat bran,
or 1 teaspoon flaxseed meal
¼ teaspoon psyllium seed powder
2 tablespoons plain yogurt
¼ teaspoon wheat germ (optional)
1 to 2 tablespoons water or juice

Combine all the ingredients in a wide-mouthed glass. Mix together lightly, adding water or juice to desired consistency. Wait a few minutes for mixture to soften before eating. Follow it with a glass of water.

Source: D. Rudin and C. Felix. *Omega-3 Oils*. Garden City Park NY: Avery Publishing Group, 1996, p. 150.

A healthy diet will usually prevent constipation. However, if you occasionally need some help, there are natural alternatives to synthetic laxatives (also see *Prescription for Nutritional Healing* in Appendix B):

- Psyllium seeds, either whole or in one of several preparations, should be taken with water.
- Karaya is a vegetable gum that should also be taken with water.
- Bentonite is ground volcanic ash that removes bacteria, parasites (see Chapter 8), and toxins from the intestinal tract. However, it can also remove probiotic bacteria and nutrients, and so it should only be used for short spans of time.
- Castor oil, elderberry, and herbal anthraquinone preparations, such as aloe and senna, all stimulate sluggish bowel muscles. Stimulant laxatives can pro-

duce side effects such as spasms and loose stools, and therefore should not be used for long periods of time.

- Coffee and lemon juice enemas, each taken once a week, will relieve constipation. Make the coffee enema by boiling six heaping tablespoons of ground coffee (not instant) in two quarts of water for fifteen minutes, cooling to a comfortable temperature, and straining. Make the lemon juice enema by adding the juice of three lemons to two quarts of lukewarm water. In both cases, use steam-distilled water to avoid introducing additional toxins into your system.[4]

Because a stressed body produces tense bowel muscles, relaxation techniques are an important part of constipation relief, in addition to their significant role in fighting mental disturbances, high blood pressure, and heart problems. Stress-reduction techniques range from long walks, meditation, massage, and exercise to reflexology, yoga, tai chi, and QiGong. For information on these techniques, look for courses and lectures at your local high school, college, or public library, or contact an alternative health practitioner in your area. Abdominal massage and deep breathing exercises are particularly soothing for bowel difficulties, especially if they are performed in front of an open window or outdoors. Remember, deep breathing uses your diaphragm, which means that your abdomen should move in and out as you breathe, and not just your chest.

RESTORING INTESTINAL HEALTH WITH WHEY

Whey is the liquid that separates out of milk as it curdles into cheese. It contains little fat and abundant amounts of protein and natural immune factors. This makes it a very beneficial substance that can restore the intestines to good health.

The Benefits of Whey

The use of whey for the relief of numerous ailments has been recommended by doctors since the time of Hippocrates. It is especially useful for overcoming septic conditions such as boils, carbuncles, and decayed teeth.[5] It appears to fight diarrhea-causing intestinal infections.[6] It is well documented as an excellent source of nutrition for premature infants.[7,8] Whey is a good supplement for athletes, given its ability to counteract muscle breakdown during strenuous activity and its concentration of amino acids that enhance muscle function.[9] Finally, whey is thought to increase life expectancy.[10,11]

Whey's benefits are derived from the nutrients it contains, including calcium and lactose, or milk sugar. Lactose nourishes the probiotic bacteria that normally inhabit the intestines, which allows the bacteria, in turn, to protect the digestive tract from disease-causing microorganisms (see Chapter 12).

Whey also contains high-quality protein. Such protein contains all of the essential amino acids, that is, those amino acids the body cannot make for itself. In fact, the protein in whey has a higher biological value than that found in eggs, which is usually considered to be the best protein.[12,13]

Whey protein consists of mainly *lactalbumin* and *lactoglobulins*, both of which enhance immunity. In one study involving mice, whey lactalbumin provided 2.4 times better immune system protection than that provided by egg protein, and five times better immune protection than casein (milk solid) protein. More importantly, this immune-stimulating effect continued when the lactalbumin was replaced by a mixture that duplicated lactalbumin's amino-acid pattern. This additional finding firmly demonstrated that the amino-acid composition of the lactalbumin found in whey is responsible for whey's effects on the immune system.[14]

Concentrated whey protein also affects levels of glutathione, probably the body's most important water-soluble antioxidant. Concentrated protein definitely raises glutathione levels in animal studies, and may do so when taken by humans.[15,16]

Ways of Using Whey

Raw whey is difficult to obtain. But powdered whey concentrate is readily available, and can be taken either as a drink or as an enema. Both provide the probiotic bacteria in the intestines with nutrients, while the enema is especially useful for intestinal cleansing.

There are a number of different whey products on the market, and a number of health practitioners have used whey to help their patients. One such practitioner is David Webster, a certified colon hygienist in Encinitas, California. He has developed the Webster Implant Technique (WIT), a rectally administered procedure that uses Kyo-Dophilus probiotic supplements and Webster's own ProFlora Whey formula, which can also be taken in drink form.[17] (See Appendix C and *Colon Flora* in Appendix B.) One of Webster's patients, a 34-year-old photographer named Richard, had suffered from daily diarrhea for the prior four months, in addition to headaches and weakness. While antibiotic therapy had provided no lasting benefits, Webster's formula, taken by mouth, stopped the diarrhea in twenty-four hours.

Molly, a 23-year-old secretary, saw Webster after suffering repeated vaginal yeast infections—a typical sign of the yeast syndrome, which starts in the intestines (see Chapter 7). The antifungal diet that Molly had followed did help, but it was so restrictive that she found it almost impossible to continue with its compliance. The diet left her underweight and excessively tired, and the over-the-counter medications she was taking had adverse side effects, too.

"I recommended that Molly douche with one tea-spoonful of Kyolic liquid garlic in four ounces of puri-fied water until her symptoms of yeast vaginitis abat-ed," Webster says. "Then she was to apply WIT. This was followed with the insertion of three capsules of Kyo-Dophilus vaginally to colonize the area with probi-otics. Using this program on a regular basis over sev-eral months, along with taking one teaspoonful of Ky-olic orally each day as a food supplement, this woman has seen no relapse for the ensuing two years."[18] For more information on the rectal implantation of probiot-ic bacteria, see Chapter 12.

Webster and other health care professionals have had good success using whey products in combination with other substances, and you may find such a program useful for your intestinal problems. However, we would urge you to not *self-diagnose* and self-treat with whey or anything else. If you have symptoms of a serious in-testinal condition (see Chapters 2 and 3), or of any other illness, you should first speak with your health care provider.

FEEDING PROBIOTIC BACTERIA WITH FOS

Research has found that a natural class of carbohydrates called fructooligosaccharides (FOS), found in a variety of foods (see Table 11.1), have the ability to selectively pro-mote the growth of friendly intestinal bacteria. FOS is used commercially as a sweetening agent, flavor en-hancer, bulking agent, and moistening substance (humec-tant). FOS is approved for human consumption in Japan, and the United States Food and Drug Administration (FDA) has approved a GRAS (generally recognized as safe) application filed by Coors Bio Tech, Inc. of West-minster, Colorado. Such an application also has been submitted to the European Economic Community for use in health foods, tabletop sweeteners, frozen desserts, dairy products, pastries, and candies. France has approved FOS as a feed supplement for pigs and rabbits.[19]

Like yogurt, FOS stimulates growth of bacteria in the lower gastrointestinal tract, passing through the upper tract unabsorbed. FOS tends to relieve constipation, suppress the production of toxins, and reduce blood glucose and cholesterol levels. Scientists have found that FOS itself causes no side effects apart from the possibility of soft stools or diarrhea and gas after ingestion of large quantities.

Table 11.1. Foods Containing FOS

FOS Content	Food
Relatively	Onion
High	Garlic
FOS	Burdock
Content	Artichoke
	Wheat
↓	Barley
	Rye
	Banana
Relatively	Asparagus
Low	Lettuce
FOS	Chicory
Content	Honey

In this chapter and throughout this book, we have discussed how probiotic bacteria are important in maintaining intestinal health. In the next chapter, we will provide a complete explanation of probiotics, and how you can use this powerful tool to both solve the problem of indigestion and improve your overall health.

CHAPTER 12

Banishing Indigestion for Good With Probiotics

Throughout this book, we have seen how much good intestinal health depends on probiotic bacteria. The term *probiotic* is taken from Greek words meaning "for life," and this term covers all of the beneficial microorganisms that make up the major portion of a healthy person's gut flora. Many of the diseases we discussed in Part One develop when conditions within the intestines fail to support these vital microbes.

Products that contain probiotic bacteria, such as yogurt and sauerkraut, have been eaten for centuries to help achieve and maintain good health and longevity. Now, both the medical community and the general public are looking for the best ways to use probiotics. In this chapter, we will explain how probiotics can improve health before telling you how to supplement your diet with these important bacteria.

POOR DIET AND INDIGESTION: BAD BACTERIA OUT OF CONTROL

When a healthy diet is followed, the billions of friendly bacteria that live in the human digestive tract outnumber the bad bacteria, 85 percent to 15 percent, and do a fine job of assisting in the assimilation of food. However, the modern diet consists of overly processed, highly sweetened, smoked, and fatty foods, all of which contain large amounts of additives. As a result, many of us eat insufficient amounts of fiber, whole grains, and raw fruits and vegetables.

As we saw in Chapter 5, the modern diet can result in dysbiosis, in which an imbalance develops between the good and bad intestinal bacteria. While good bacteria thrive in the acid environment found in a healthy intestinal tract, bad bacteria prefer the alkaline environment created by a poor diet. Dysbiosis can lead to digestive tract disorders and symptoms, such as heartburn, gas, bloating, irritable bowel syndrome, diarrhea, constipation, and cold sores, as well as disorders elsewhere in the body, including vaginal and urinary tract infections.

Dysbiosis can also lead to a condition known as *intestinal toxemia*. Sometimes referred to as autointoxication, intestinal toxemia occurs when the body is poisoned by wastes derived from improper digestion. Symptoms of intestinal toxemia include:[1]

- Digestive disorders, such as bloating, gas, diarrhea, constipation, and abdominal cramps

- Chronic fatigue

- Depression

- Anxiety attacks

- Frequent colds and sinus infections

- Skin disorders, such as eczema, pimples, rashes, and itching

- Loss of libido

- Premenstrual syndrome

Unfortunately, many people treat the symptoms of indigestion without treating its root causes. Led on by a bombardment of advertising, they take a variety of non-prescription antacids and H2 blockers. These drugs are themselves harmful to health, and can produce symptoms such as constipation, heartburn, chest pain, and gas (see Chapter 1). As a result, the basic problem is not addressed, and a number of years may elapse before a person becomes aware of the damage that has been done.

PROBIOTICS: THE GOOD BACTERIA TAKE CHARGE

Jeffrey Moss, D.D.S., C.N.S., C.C.N., a wholistic nutrition writer, describes the gut flora as "an ever faithful, vigilant watchdog standing guard at the primary barrier that separates us from a universe of hostile factors."[2] This watchdog is made up of several pounds of microorganisms, spread among at least several hundred species. Despite the huge number of individual microbes, a healthy gut flora acts in unison to process food and protect the digestive tract. These bacteria, called *resident bacteria*, occupy a limited number of living spaces along the intestinal walls. The optimum situation is for most of the available spaces to be filled with beneficial bacteria: More friendly organisms means less space for harmful ones. Some kinds of good bacteria, called *transient bacteria*, do not stay in the intestines, but instead pass through them. Both resident and transient probiotics are required for good digestion (see *Probiotics* in Appendix B).

Of all the species of probiotic bacteria found within the digestive tract, three are especially important: *Lactobacillus acidophilus, Bifidobacterium bifidum*, and *Bifidobac-*

terium longum. These microbes produce a number of substances, including acetic acid, that protect the system against disease-promoting organisms. *L. acidophilus,* aided by another organism called *Streptococcus thermophilus,* predominates in the upper small intestine, while the two bifidobacteria species dominate the lower small intestine and the large intestine. When taken in supplement form together, they protect the entire intestinal tract.[3-5] Collectively, these bacteria aid digestion in a number of ways:

- They promote the development of enzymes that assist in the digestion of protein and fat.[6,7]

- They normalize the bowel's action and increase the speed at which food passes through the system.[8]

- They reduce the amount of gas produced by the intestines.[9]

- They aid in the digestion of lactose, or milk sugar, which counteracts the gas, bloating, and cramps produced by lactose intolerance (see Chapter 1).[10,11]

- They manufacture several of the B vitamins, including riboflavin, cobalamin, thiamin, folic acid, and pantothenic acid, along with some amino acids.[12-15]

- They prevent the overgrowth of *Candida albicans,* and thus suppress the yeast syndrome, which often produces digestive problems (see Chapter 7).

The importance of probiotic bacteria and the substances they produce can be seen in the fact that the numbers of beneficial bacteria found in healthy adults far exceed those found in sick or elderly people. Many illnesses may be influenced, not by the presence of a specific disease-causing agent, but rather by the absence of normal intestinal flora.[16]

PROBIOTICS FOR OVERALL HEALTH

It is not surprising that probiotics have such a positive effect on intestinal health, but there is more to it than that. The presence of probiotic bacteria benefits the entire body by promoting overall health in a number of ways:

- Natural antibiotics are produced, and about two dozen disease-causing microorganisms are inhibited.[17-20]

- Urinary tract and vaginal infections are reduced or eliminated.[21-23]

- The immune system is strengthened.[24-29]

- Some probiotic bacteria can neutralize carcinogenic, or cancer-causing, substances (see page 135). These bacteria also exhibit general antitumor properties.[30,31]

- Bifidobacteria cause a decrease in excessive cholesterol production, thus reducing the risk of atherosclerosis, or hardening of the arteries, and heart disease.[32-35]

- *L. acidophilus* hinders the production of hazardous substances, such as ammonia, indole, and hydrogen sulfide. The presence of bifidobacteria enhance this effect, and the combination of probiotic strains tends to reduce the incidence of liver disease.[36-38]

- Certain skin disorders, such as atopic dermatitis, heal more readily.[39]

Many people have found relief from a variety of ills through probiotic supplementation. Ben, a 32-year-old accountant from Alabama, had suffered from chronic mouth ulcers caused by oral herpes since childhood. Intense pain had made eating difficult, and he had lost weight. One doctor prescribed Zovirax, a powerful antiviral drug, but the ulcers only became worse. Meanwhile, Ben experimented with various brands of probiotic supplements, looking for a permanent solution to his problem. He eventually settled on Kyo-Dophilus, and found that his ulcers finally disappeared.

In Chapter 7, we saw how probiotics could help people with the yeast syndrome. Now let us take a closer look at how probiotics can help fight chronic fatigue syndrome and cancer.

Probiotics and Chronic Fatigue Syndrome

Chronic fatigue and immune dysfunction syndrome (CFIDS) is a debilitating disease that has affected millions of people around the world. Its most notable symptom is an overwhelming, draining fatigue not associated with any other known cause. Other symptoms include depression and/or anxiety plus a number of flu-like complaints, including sore throat, headache, painful lymph nodes, muscle weakness or pain, and mild fever. While doctors are not yet sure of what causes CFIDS, they believe it occurs in people whose immune systems have been weakened by stressors associated with modern life, such as poor eating habits, toxic overload from food additives and pollution, and alcohol and drug use.[40] This immune system weakness in turn allows a number of viruses, bacteria, and parasites to grow unchecked. (For more information on CFIDS, see *The Downhill Syndrome* and *From Fatigued to Fantastic!* in Appendix C.)

Because CFIDS is a complex of various disorders and symptom groups, each patient needs to follow a detailed, individualized treatment plan. Probiotic supplementation is an important part of a good CFIDS treatment plan because it can help fight several of the disorders associated with chronic fatigue, including food allergies and the leaky gut syndrome (Chapter 6), and the yeast syndrome (Chapter 7).

Lois, a 44-year-old real estate broker in Washington state, had seen her life nearly ruined by CFIDS: lost jobs, thousands of dollars in medical bills, the inability to care for her children, and even several suicide attempts. The massive doses of antibiotics that she had taken killed the good bacteria in her intestines, and she suffered from yeast vaginitis, a symptom of the yeast syndrome, as well as sinus infections, canker sores, and constipation. Finally, Lois found a successful treatment program, one that included the regular consumption of yogurt (see Chapter 10) and a probiotic supplement taken both orally and as a vaginal suppository. The probiotic helped to both eliminate the CFIDS itself and put an end to all her other symptoms. As a result, Lois enjoyed "a boundless energy" that she had never experienced before.

Probiotics and Cancer

Cancer is one of the industrialized world's most dreaded diseases, and with good reason: Both the incidence of cancer and its associated death rate continue to rise, despite all the time and money spent on searching for a cure. In 1996, there were 1.3 million new cases of solid tumor malignancy, lymphoma, and blood dyscrasia in the United States,[41] and cancer is soon expected to overtake heart disease as the most frequent killer of North Americans.

The World Health Organization, backed up by the United States Department of Health and Human Services along with the National Academy of Sciences, estimates that more than 80 percent of all cancer cases result from exposure to carcinogens that are all around us—at home, at work, at play, at the dinner table, and in nearly every other area of daily life. "An ounce of prevention is worth a pound of cure" is nowhere so true as with cancer. It is important to find substances that can protect us against the roughly 105,000 common cancer-causing agents now being produced in industrialized countries.[42]

Among the worst and most common of these carcinogens are the *nitrosamines*. These chemicals are created when the food additive sodium nitrite interacts with normal protein breakdown products called secondary amines. Amines are also produced when juices from poultry, seafood, or meat are broken down by high heat.[43] Secondary amines, especially dimethylamine and morpholine, are virtually everywhere in our environment. They exist in relatively high concentrations in many fast foods, such as French fries, hamburgers, and fried chicken, and in smoked meats and fish, such as hot dogs, bacon, and lox. Dozens of other foods contain lower concentrations. Nitrosamines are also used in industrial processes of all types, including those used to make pesticides and drugs. They are produced by internal combustion engines, and therefore exist in the air we breathe. Finally, nitrosamines are present in cigarette smoke, including secondhand smoke breathed in by nonsmokers, and have helped to make lung cancer one of the most common of all malignancies.[44] Even in low doses, nitrosamines encourage other weak carcinogens to increase their cancer-causing potential.[45]

Probiotic bacteria detoxify nitrosamines within the intestines, thereby making probiotic supplementation a powerful weapon in the battle against cancer. The ability of probiotic bacteria to fight cancer has been shown in experiments by Tomotari Mitsuoka, Ph.D., Professor of Biomedical Science at the University of Tokyo. Dr. Mitsuoka used mice that possessed large amounts of friendly bacteria and no harmful intestinal flora of any type, and that ordinarily were predisposed to developing liver cancer. When compared with similar mice who had a normal mix of beneficial and harmful organisms, the germ-free mice experienced much lower cancer rates—39 percent to 85 percent. However, when the germ-free mice were exposed to various strains of disease-causing bacteria and bred, their offspring experienced much higher cancer rates—up to 100 percent, in some cases—depending on the specific type of bacteria introduced.[46]

Dr. Mitsuoka reported another highly significant finding. When *L. acidophilus* was used in combination with different types of disease-causing bacteria, the incidence of liver cancer was reduced by 40 percent when compared with animals without any lactobacilli. This discovery suggests that lactobacilli detoxify substances produced by other bacteria.

The ability of friendly bacteria to detoxify cancer-causing agents in the human intestine has also been demonstrated.[47] There are several enzymes within the stool that can promote the development of cancer, and strict vegetarians have lower levels of these enzymes than do people who eat meat.[48] However, feeding lactobacilli to meat-eaters reduces their harmful-enzyme levels to those seen in vegetarians.[49] This makes the regular use of probiotic supplements an important part of an overall cancer-fighting strategy.

GETTING THE PROBIOTICS YOU NEED

Humans have intuitively understood the need for a healthy gut flora even before anyone knew that microbes existed. Ancient peoples, including the entire Roman Empire as well as the army of Ghengis Khan, habitually consumed cultured foods with every meal. In the eighteenth century, the seamen who served with

Dutch trans-Atlantic explorers ate cultured foods. So did sailors in the British Navy, thanks to Dr. James Lind, who came up with the idea of fermenting sauerkraut in wooden barrels aboard ship. Miso, or fermented soybean paste, is a traditional Japanese staple.

Today, sauerkraut is consumed in quantity by Germans, fermented vegetables are enjoyed by Asians, and yogurt is enjoyed by various peoples around the globe. Probiotics have also recently become popular as food supplements. These supplements usually come in the form of capsules, tablets, tinctures (concentrated liquids in alcohol), or powders.

Not all probiotic supplements are equally effective, for a variety of reasons, and you have to experiment to see which brand works best for you. As we have seen, digestive health depends on a number of probiotic species, especially *L. acidophilus, B. longum,* and *B. bifidum,* and not on any one type of bacteria. All these organisms work together to aid digestion and protect against disease. The bifidobacteria are particularly important to the health of the large intestine, which is where digestive problems occur in many people. Thus, the most effective probiotic supplements contain a mix of bacteria.[50]

The medical community now recognizes that while many probiotic species live within many different types of hosts, each species adapts to each particular host in a slightly different way. For example, lactobacilli taken from one host will not take up residence within another. Therefore, probiotics used for human consumption should themselves have originated from humans.

To be effective, probiotic supplements must be carefully manufactured. The following production factors are crucial:

• There must be enough organisms—about 1.5 billion in each dose—to provide the desired effect, and these organisms must be genetically uniform from batch to batch.

- Manufacturing conditions must be scrupulously clean, not only to avoid contamination but to make the final product as allergy-free as possible.

- The supplement must be heat stable, which both eliminates the need for refrigeration and gives the product a long shelf life.

How you take a probiotic supplement is as important as which brand you choose. Some people believe that you should consume live cultures on an empty stomach. This is incorrect! In almost all situations, it's best to take probiotics during a meal or within forty-five minutes afterwards, as food effectively makes the stomach more alkaline, or higher in pH, than usual. At this higher pH, the fragile dried probiotics have a greater chance of survival as they pass to the small intestine—probiotic bacteria prefer an acidic environment, but the stomach is normally too acidic. In addition, the stomach empties rapidly right after a meal, which further minimizes the bacteria's exposure to damaging gastric juices.

Oral probiotic supplements can often prevent intestinal problems from occurring, and can even help cure existing disorders. If you need a little more help, though, you may want to try rectal probiotic implantation. One homeopathic physician who uses this method, Abram Ber, M.D., of Phoenix, tests each patient to determine which species can help that person, and what dosage is needed. He then employs the services of a trained implantation specialist, who introduces the probiotics into the patient's large intestine through the rectum. Ber says, "Never have I seen a treatment . . . render so much benefit to so many people. This is definitely a therapeutic advancement."[51] (For more information, see Chapter 11.)

We would strongly urge you to make probiotics a part of your daily routine, and clear all the antacids, H2 blockers, antinausea drugs, and other pills and potions out of your medicine cabinet. Probiotics can not only banish indigestion, but can also make a real difference in your overall health and well-being. In the next chapter, we will leave you with some parting thoughts.

Conclusion

As we have seen, a long-term solution to heartburn and other digestive ills does not come out of a bottle. Rather, treating and preventing indigestion involves taking good care of one's probiotic bacteria, those tiny creatures that promote both good digestion and strong immune defenses. A healthy person's intestinal walls are coated with billions of both healthful and harmful bacteria. The healthful bacteria filter out damaging substances, such as viruses, disease-causing bacteria, fungi, toxins, and wastes, while allowing nutrients and water to be absorbed. Health writer Dr. Jeffrey Moss calls these bacteria, known as the gut flora, an "organ-within-an-organ," and says, "the symbiotic relationship that we have with this world within us should not be an afterthought, as it often is."[1]

Microbiologists agree that other things being equal, each person's health depends upon the kind of flora dominating his or her intestines. "Show me an individual who has retained the natural [*Lactobacillus*] *acidophilus* bacillus of childhood," says one veteran microbiologist, "and I will show you a healthy man or woman." Unfortunately, life in the modern industrialized world often leads to an imbalance between probiotic and disease-causing bacteria, with the result that many people suffer from chronic digestive problems. A diet that is high in fat and low in fiber, combined with smoking, stress, excessive alcohol consumption, and the overuse of medications such as antacids and painkillers, favors the growth and spread of bad microbes. Another distressing practice—perhaps one of the worst—is the overuse of broad-spectrum antibiotics (see page 53). Researchers have acknowledged that virtually every antibiotic taken orally causes alterations in the balance of the bacteria within the intestines. Just one course of medication may upset the composition of the gut flora, reducing the individual's resistance to intestinal and systemic ill health.

Restoring intestinal health first requires a change in diet, with a reduction in or elimination of highly processed, sugary, and fatty foods, and a corresponding increase in whole grains, fresh fruits and vegetables, limited amounts of organically raised meat, and cultured foods such as yogurt. These changes in diet must be supported by adequate exercise, rest, and stress reduction. If constipation or other large-intestine disorders are present, internal cleansers can restore regularity.

Finally, the permanent banishment of indigestion requires the daily use of probiotic supplements. The benefits provided by probiotics go beyond aiding the digestive process. They include helping the body fight disorders such as the yeast syndrome and chronic fatigue, and even extend to cancer prevention.

The work of Elie Metchnikoff, the Russian bacteriologist who first explained the idea of intestinal imbalance, has been largely ignored among gastroenterologists practicing conventional medicine in the United States and Canada. But it has influenced four generations of European physicians, and throughout nearly all of Europe, the use of probiotics is highly popular. It is important for doctors to stop focusing on assigning labels to a patient's disease, such as "irritable bowel syndrome" or "ulcerative colitis," and to instead concentrate on both the symptoms and the underlying dysfunction these symptoms represent. There are signs that conventional doctors are at least starting to go beyond the drugs-and-surgery approach to chronic digestive disorders. As a result, there are growing numbers of doctors who use alternative treatment approaches to these common problems.

Doctors are starting to take alternative treatments seriously because significant numbers of laypeople are turning away from over-the-counter medications, and are looking for more natural methods of heartburn and indigestion relief. The power to improve your digestive health lies within your reach. It starts with self-education, through books such as this one and those listed in Appendix B. If you already suffer from a serious intestinal disorder, your need for knowledge is even more urgent—do not be afraid to question your doctor about his or her recommendations. Then make the necessary changes in your lifestyle, including the regular use of probiotic supplements. You will reap a lifetime of good health.

APPENDIX A

Resource List

Obviously, your first source of information about digestive diseases should be your doctor or other health care provider. However, there are organizations, listed below, that you can contact for additional information about specific problems.

American Academy of Pediatrics (AAP)
141 Northwest Point Boulevard
P.O. Box 927
Elk Grove Village IL 60009-0927
(800) 433-9016

**American Association for the Study
of Liver Diseases (AASLD)**
Slac Inc.
6900 Grove Road
Thorofair NJ 08086
(609) 848-1000

American Board of Pediatrics (ABP)
111 Silver Cedar Court
Chapel Hill NC 27514
(919) 929-0461

American Celiac Society
58 Musano Court
West Orange NJ 07052
(201) 325-8837

American Gastroenterological Association (AGA)
6900 Grove Road
Thorofair NJ 08086
(609) 848-1000

American Hospital Association (AHA)
1 North Franklin
Chicago IL 60606
(312) 422-3000

American Liver Foundation
1425 Pompton Avenue
Cedar Grove NJ 07009
(973) 857-2626

**American Society of Colon and
   Rectal Surgeons (ASCRS)**
85 West Algonquin Road
Suite 550
Arlington Heights IL 60005
(847) 290-9184

The Bockus International Society of Gastroenterology
398 Donenech Avenue
Hata Rey PR 00918
(787) 764-8787

Cystic Fibrosis Foundation (CF Foundation)
6931 Arlington Boulevard
Bethesda MD 20814
(301) 770-1682

Dean Thiel Foundation (DTF)
1425 Pompton Avenue
Cedar Grove NJ 07009
(973) 857-2626
(see the American Liver Foundation)

Digestive Diseases Clearinghouse,
  the National Institute of Arthritis, Diabetes,
  and Digestive and Kidney Diseases (NIADDK)
National Institutes of Health
9000 Rockville Pike
Bethesda MD 20892
(301) 496-4000

The Gail I. Zuckerman Foundation
2600 Netherland Avenue
Riverdale NY 10463
(212) 884-7950

The Gastro-Intestinal Research Foundation (GIRF)
70 East Lake Street
Suite 1015
Chicago IL 60601
(312) 332-1350

International Association for Enterostomal Therapy, Inc.
505 North Tustin, Suite 282
Santa Ana CA 92705
(714) 972-1720

Iron Overload Diseases Association, Inc. (IOD)
433 Westwind Drive
North Palm Beach FL 33408
(561) 840-8512

National Foundation for Ileitis and Colitis
386 Park Avenue South
New York NY 10016
(212) 685-3440

**The North American Society
  for Pediatric Gastroenterology**
Children's Hospital Research Foundation
33 Burnet Avenue
Cincinnati OH 45229
(513) 636-4238

Reach Out for Youth With Ileitis and Colitis
15 Chemung Place
Jericho NY 11753
(516) 822-8010

**Society of American Gastrointestinal
  Endoscopic Surgeons (SAGES)**
Thomas Jefferson University Hospital
111 South Eleventh Street
Philadelphia PA 19107
(215) 955-6000

United Ostomy Association
36 Executive Park
Suite 120
Irvine CA 92714
(800) 826-0826

APPENDIX B

Suggested Reading List

Colon Flora: The Missing Link in Immunity, Health & Longevity. D. Webster. Cardiff CA: Hygeia Publishing, 1995.

The Downhill Syndrome. P. Yutsis and M. Walker. Garden City Park NY: Avery Publishing Group, 1997.

From Fatigued to Fantastic! J. Teitelbaum. Garden City Park NY: Avery Publishing Group, 1996.

The Green Tea Book. L.A. Mitscher and V. Dolby. Garden City Park NY: Avery Publishing Group, 1998.

Guess What Came to Dinner: Parasites and Your Health. A.L. Gittleman. Garden City Park: Avery Publishing Group, 1993.

Hidden Food Allergies. S. Astor. Garden City Park NY: Avery Publishing Group, 1997.

Indigestion: Living Better with Upper Intestinal Problems From Heartburn to Ulcers and Gallstones. H.D. Janowitz. New York: Oxford University Press, 1992.

Omega 3 Oils. D. Rudin and C. Felix. Garden City Park NY: Avery Publishing Group, 1996.

Prescription for Nutritional Healing. J.F. Balch and P.A. Balch. 2nd ed. Garden City Park NY: Avery Publishing Group, 1997.

Probiotics. N. Trenev. Garden City Park NY: Avery Publishing Group, 1998.

7 Weeks to a Settled Stomach. R.L. Hoffman. New York: Pocket Books, 1990.

The Ultimate Nutrient: Glutamine. J. Shabert and N. Ehrlich. Garden City Park NY: Avery Publishing Group, 1994.

When Antibiotics Fail. M. Lappe'. Berkeley CA: North Atlantic Books, 1995.

The Yeast Connection. W.G. Crook. 3rd ed. Jackson MS: Professional Books, 1986.

The Yeast Syndrome. J.P. Trowbridge and M. Walker. New York: Bantam Books, 1986.

Yeast-Related Illnesses. J.P. Trowbridge and M. Walker. Greenwich CT: Devin-Adair Publishers, 1987.

Your Gut Feelings. H.D. Janowitz. New York: Oxford University Press, 1994.

APPENDIX C

Sources of Products and Services

Fiber Supplements

Aerobic Bulk Cleanse (ABC)
Aerobic Life Industries
3045 South 46th Street
Phoenix AZ 85040
800-798-0707
602-968-0707

A.M./P.M. Ultimate Cleanse
Nature's Secret
5485 Conestoga Court
Boulder CO 80301
800-525-9696
303-546-6306

Garlic Supplements

Kyolic
Wakunaga of America Company, Ltd.
23501 Madero
Mission Viejo CA 92691-2764
800-421-2998
714-855-2776

Herbal Antiparasitic Formulas

Paracan-144
ParaMycocidin
Allergy Research Group
Nutricology, Inc.
Stephen A. Levine, Ph.D.
P.O. Box 489
San Leandro CA 94577-0489
800-545-9960
510-639-4572
Fax: 510-635-6730

Parasitology

Great Smokies Diagnostic Laboratory
President Stephen Barrie
Laboratory Director Martin Lee
63 Zillicoa Street
Asheville NC 28801-1084
800-522-4762
704-253-0621

Probiotic Supplements

Kyo-Dophilus
Wakunaga of America Company, Ltd.
23501 Madero
Mission Viejo CA 92691-2764
800-421-2998
714-855-2776

Soy Beverages

Haelan 851
The Haelan Products Group
Metaire LA
800-542-3526

Yogurt Manufacturers

Butterworks Farm
Westfield VT 05874

Natural Horizons, Inc.
Boulder CO 80301

Seven Stars Farm, Inc.
Phoenixville PA 19460

Stonyfield Farm
Londonderry NH 03053

Notes

Introduction

1. Hoffman R.L. *7 Weeks to a Settled Stomach*. New York: Pocket Books, 1990, p. 137.

2. Trowbridge J.P. and Walker M. *The Yeast Syndrome*. New York: Bantam Books, 1986, pp. 158–160.

CHAPTER 1

The Size of the Indigestion Problem

1. Profile of consumers in need. *Progressive Grocer,* September 1995, pp. 98–99.

2. Freudenheim M. War on heartburn heats up with over-the-counter blitz. *The New York Times,* 8 September 1995, p. 1.

3. When it's not an ulcer. *Consumer Reports,* August 1995, p. 552.

4. Antacids: which beat heartburn best? *Consumer Reports,* July 1994, p. 444.

5. Antacids: which beat heartburn best? *Consumer Reports,* July 1994, pp. 444–445.

6. Mindell E. Top-secret natural remedies—far superior to "wonder drugs!" Tri-Cities WA: Alpha EnterPrises, 3 December 1995, Plan B E-mail, DoPlanB@aol.com.

CHAPTER 2

Problems in the Upper Digestive Tract

1. Powell L.W. and Pipe D.W. (eds). *Fundamentals of Gastroenterology.* 6th ed. Sydney: McGraw-Hill Book Co., 1995, p. 3.

2. William Perlow, interviewed by Morton Walker.

3. Janowitz H.D. *Indigestion: Living Better with Upper Intestinal Problems From Heartburn to Ulcers and Gallstones.* New York: Oxford University Press, 1992, p. 79.

4. Janowitz H.D. *Indigestion: Living Better with Upper Intestinal Prblems from Heartburn to Ulcers and Gallstones.* New York: Oxford University Press, 1992, p. 195.

5. National Digestive Diseases Education and Information Clearinghouse. *Cirrhosis of the liver.* DD Clearinghouse Fact Sheet. Public Health Service, NIH: U.S. Department of Health and Human Services, 1989.

6. National Institute of Arthritis, Diabetes, Digestive and Kidney Diseases. *What is pancreatitis?* NIADDK Fact Sheet. Public Health Service, NIH: U.S. Department of Health and Human Services, 1988.

CHAPTER 3

Problems in the Lower Digestive Tract

1. Fisher R.L. (ed). Malabsorption and nutritional status and support. *Gastroenterology Clinics of North America,* 18, 1989.

2. Hoffman R.L. *7 Weeks to a Settled Stomach.* New York: Pocket Books, 1990, p. 133.

3. Don't drink to this. *Nutrition Action Healthletter* 22(5):10, 1995.

4. Sleisenger M.H. and Fordtran J.S. (eds). *Gastrointestinal Disease: Pathophysiology, Diagnosis and Management.* 5th ed. Philadelphia: W.B. Saunders, 1993.

5. Janowitz H.D. *Your Gut Feelings.* New York: Oxford University Press, 1994, p. 43.

6. Fiber 1, diverticulosis 0. *Nutrition Action Healthletter* 22(1):2, 1995.

7. Chaitow L. and Trenev N. *Probiotics: The Revolutionary, "Friendly Bacteria" Way to Vital Health and Well-being.* Northamptonshire, England: Thorsons Publishing Group, 1990, pp. 28, 29–30.

8. Doe W. F. The immunology of the gut. In Lachmann P.J., Peters D.K., Rosen F.S., and Walport M. (eds): *Clinical Aspects of Immunology*, 4th ed. Sidney: Blackwells, 1993, pp. 2079–2090.

9. Janowitz H.D. *Your Gut Feelings.* New York: Oxford University Press, 1994, p. 24.

10. Hoffman R.L. *7 Weeks to a Settled Stomach.* New York: Pocket Books, 1990, p. 220.

11. Hoffman R.L. *7 Weeks to a Settled Stomach.* New York: Pocket Books, 1990, p. 221.

12. Heidl R. Isotherapy of haemorrhoidal complaints: widespread affliction has good therapy chances. *Explore* 6(6): 18–21, 1996.

CHAPTER 4
Fighting the Bacteria That Cause Ulcers

1. Marshall B.J. and Warren J.R. Unidentified curved bacillus on gastric epithelium in active chronic gastritis. *Lancet* 1:1273–1275, 1983.

2. Marshall B.J. and others. Unidentified curved bacilli in the stomach of patients with gastritis and peptic ulceration. *Lancet* I:1311, 1984.

3. Marshall B.J. and others. Attempt to fulfill Koch's postulates for *Helicobacter pylori*. *Medical Journal of Australia* 42:436, 1985.

4. Dooley C.P. Background and historical considerations of *Helicobacter pylori*. *Gastroenterology Clinics of North America* 22(1):1–4, 1993.

5. *Nutrition Action Healthletter* 23(8):3, 1996.

6. Marshall B. *Helicobacter pylori*. In: *Dysbiosis: A Clinical Symposium.* Asheville NC: Great Smokies Diagnostic Laboratory, 1992.

7. Freudenheim M. Drug companies discount ulcer treatment advice. *The New York Times*, 10 February 1994, p. D21.

8. Kolata G. New study backs ulcer-cure theory. *The New York Times*, 6 May 1992.

9. Balch J.F. and Balch P.A. *Prescription for Nutritional Healing*. 2nd ed. Garden City Park NY: Avery Publishing Group, 1997, p. 425.

10. Altman L.K. Antimicrobial drugs endorsed for ulcers in a major U.S. shift. *The New York Times*, 10 February 1994, p. 1.

11. Wade N. Scientists map a bacterium's genetic code. *The New York Times*, 7 August 1997, p. B8.

12. Walsh J.H. Editorial. *Annals of Internal Medicine* May 1992.

13. *Helicobacer pylori Detection*. Asheville NC: Great Smokies Diagnostic Laboatory, 1992, p. 4.

14. Noble W.C. Skin as a microbial habitat. In de Louvois J. (ed): *Selected Topics in Clinical Bacteriology*. Baltimore: Williams & Wilkins, 1976, pp. 235–256.

15. Mackowiak P.A. The normal microbial flora. *New England Journal of Medicine* 307(2):83–93, 1982.

16. Does fiber foil ulcers? *Nutrition Action Healthletter* 24(4):14, 1997.

Inset: The Dangers of Antibiotics

1. Lappe' M. *When Antibiotics Fail*. Berkeley CA: North Atlantic Books, 1995.

2. Garrett L. A bacterial breeding ground. *Newsday*, 28 October 1997, pp. C4–C9.

3. Alleger I. Too much of a good thing. *Townsend Letter for Doctors & Patients*, January 1996, p. 128.

4. McKenna J. *Alternatives to Antibiotics*. Dublin: Gill & Macmillan Ltd, 1996, pp. 29, 37.

CHAPTER 5

How Bad Bacteria Can Harm the Intestines

1. Brown J.P. Role of gut bacterial flora in nutrition and health: A review of recent advances in bacteriological tech-

niques, metabolism and factors affecting flora composition. *CRC Reviews in Food Science and Nutrition* 8:229–336, 1977.

2. Brown J.P. Role of gut bacterial flora in nutrition and health: a review of recent advances in bacteriological techniques, metabolism and factors affecting flora composition. *CRC Reviews in Food Science and Nutrition* 8:229–336, 1977.

3. Berghouse L., Hori S., Hill M., Hudson M., Lennard-Jones J.E., and Rogers E. Comparison between the bacterial and oligosaccharide content of ileostomy effluent in subjects taking diets rich in refined or unrefined carbohydrate. *Gut* 25:1071–1077, 1984.

4. Haenel H. and Bendig J. Intestinal flora in health and disease. *Progress in Food and Nutrition Science* 1: 21–64, 1975.

5. Kistler L.A. and Gianella R.A. Relationship of intestinal bacteria to malabsorption. *Practical Gastroenterology* 4:24–44, 1980.

6. Bennet J.D. Ulcerative colitis: the result of an altered bacterial metabolism of bile acids or cholesterol. *Medical Hypotheses* 20:125–132, 1986.

7. Alun Jones V., Shorthouse M., McLaughlin P., Workman E., and Hunter J.O. Food intolerance: a major factor in the pathogenesis of irritable bowel syndrome. *Lancet* 2: 1115–1117, 1980.

8. Bayliss C.E., Bradley H.K., Alun Jones V., and Hunter J.O. Some aspects of colonic microbial activity in irritable bowel syndrome associated with food intolerance. *Annali dell Instituto superiore di Sanita* 22:959–964, 1986.

9. Hunter J.O. and Alun Jones V. Studies on the pathogenesis of irritable bowel syndrome produced by food intolerance. In Read N.W. (ed): *The Irritable Bowel Syndrome*. New York: Grune and Stratton, 1985, pp. 185–190.

10. Beeken W.L. Remedial defects in Crohn's disease. *Archives Internal Medicine* 135:686–690, 1975.

11. Serrander R., Magnusson K.E., Kihlstrom E., and Sundqvist T. Acute yersinia infections in man increase intestinal permeability for low-molecular weight polyethylene glycols

(PEG 400). *Scandinavian Journal of Infectious Disease* 18(5): 409–413, 1986.

12. Hollander D., Vadheim C., Brettholz E., Petersen G.M., Delahunty T., and Rotter J.I. Increased intestinal permeability in patients with Crohn's disease and their relatives. *Annals Internal Medicine* 105:883–885, 1986.

13. Lictman S.N., Keku J., Schwab J.H., and Sartor R.B. Hepatic injury associated with small bowel bacterial overgrowth in rats is prevented by metronidazole and tetracycline. *Gastroenterology* 100:513–519, 1991.

14. Ionescu G., Kiehl R., Ona L., and Schuler R. Abnormal fecal microflora and malabsorption phenomena in atopic eczema patients. *Journal of Advancement in Medicine* 3:71–89, 1990.

15. Ionescu G., Kiehl R., Wichmann-Kunz F., and Leimbeck R. Immunobiological significance of fungal and bacterial infections in atopic eczema. *Journal of Advancement in Medicine* 3:47–58, 1990.

16. Newmark H.L. and Lupton J.R. Determinants and consequences of colonic luminal pH: implications for colon cancer. *Nutrition and Cancer* 14:161–173, 1990.

17. Malhotra S.L. Fecal urobilingen levels and pH of stools. *Journal of the Royal Society of Medicine* 75:710, 1982.

18. Chung K.T., Fulk G.E., and Slein M.W. Tryptophanase of fecal flora as a possible factor in the etiology of colon cancer. *Journal of the National Cancer Institute* 54:1073–1078, 1975.

19. Goldin B.R. The metabolism of the intestinal microflora and its relationship to dietary fat, colon and breast cancer. In: *Dietary Fat and Cancer*. New York: Alan R. Liss, 1986, pp. 655–685.

20. Hill M.J., Melviulle D.M., Lennard-Jones J.E., Neale K., and Ritchie J.K. Faecal bile acids, dysplasia, and carcinoma in ulcerative colitis. *Lancet* 2:185–186, 1987.

21. Bennet J.D. Ulcerative colitis: the result of an altered bacterial metabolism of bile acids or cholesterol. *Medical Hypotheses* 20:125–132, 1986.

22. Baker S. Introductory comments. In: *Dysbiosis: A Clinical*

Symposium. Asheville NC: Great Smokies Diagnostic Laboratory, 1992, p. 1–4.

23. Baker S. Introductory comments. In: *Dysbiosis: A Clinical Symposium.* Asheville NC: Great Smokies Diagnostic Laboratory, 1992, p. 1–4.

24. Burnhill M. Vaginal dysbiosis. In: *Dysbiosis: A Clinical Symposium.* Asheville NC: Great Smokies Diagnostic Laboratory, 1992, pp. 11–13.

CHAPTER 6
Poor Digestion and the Leaky Gut Syndrome

1. Lahasmaa-Rantala R. and others. Intestinal permeability in patients with yersinia triggered reactive arthritis. *Annals of Rheumatic Disease* 50(2):91–94, 1991.

2. Serrander R., Magnusson K.E., and Sundqvist T. Acute infections with *Giardia lamblia* and rotavirus decrease intestinal permeability to low-molecular weight polyethylene glycols (PEG 400). *Scandinavian Journal of Infectious Disease* 16(4):339–344, 1984.

3. Serrander, R., Magnusson K.E., Kihlstrom E., and Sundqvist T. Acute yersinia infections in man increase intestinal permeability for low-molecular weight polyethylene glycols (PEG 400). *Scandinavian Journal of Infectious Disease* 18(5): 409–413, 1986.

4. Lim S.G. and others. Intestinal permeability and function in patients infected with human immunodeficiency virus. A comparison with coeliac disease. *Scandinavian Journal of Gastroenterology* 28(7):573–580, 1993.

5. Bjarnason I., Wise R., and Peters T. The leaky gut of alcoholism: possible route of entry for toxic compounds. *Lancet* I:79–82, 1984.

6. Worthington B.S., Meserole L., and Syrotuck J.A. Effect of daily ethanol ingestion on intestinal permeability to macromolecules. *American Journal of Digestive Disease* 23(1):23–32, 1978.

7. Jenkins R.T. and others. Increased intestinal permeability

in patients with rheumatoid arthritis: a side-effect of oral nonsteroidal anti-inflammatory drug therapy? *British Journal of Rheumatology* 26(2):103–107, 1987.

8. Bjarnason I. and others. Effect of non-steroidal anti-inflammatory drugs on the human small intestine. *Drugs* 1:35–41, 1986.

9. Rooney P.J. and Jenkins R.T. Nonsteroidal anti-inflammatory drugs (NSAIDs) and the bowel mucosa: changes in intestinal permeability may not be due to changes in prostaglandins. Letter. *Clinical Experiments in Rheumatology* 8(3):328–329, 1990.

10. Bjarnason, I. and others. Intestinal permeability to 51 Cr-EDTA in rats with experimentally induced enteropathy. *Gut* 26(6):579–585, 1985.

11. Lifschitz C.H. and Mahoney D.H. Low-dose methotrexate-induced changes in intestinal permeability determined by polyethylene glycol polymers. *Journal of Pediatric Gastroenterology Nutrition* 9(3): 301–306, 1989.

12. Berg R.D. The translocation of the normal flora bacteria from the gastrointestinal tract to the mesenteric lymph nodes and other organs. *Microecology Therapy* 11:27–34, 1981.

13. Ohri S.K. and others. Cardiopulmonary bypass impairs small intestinal transport and increases gut permeability. *Annals of Thoracic Surgery* 55(5):1080–1086, 1993.

14. Ohri S.K. and others. The effect of intestinal hypoperfusion on intestinal absorption and permeability during cardiopulmonary bypass. *Gastroenterology* 106(2):318–323, 1994.

15. Marston W. Gut reactions. *Newsweek*, 17 November 1997, pp. 95, 99.

16. Katz K.D. and others. Intestinal permeability in patients with Crohn's disease and their healthy relatives. *Gastroenterology* 97(4):927–931, 1989.

17. Pearson A.D. and others. Intestinal permeability in children with Crohn's disease and coeliac disease. *British Medical Journal* 285(6334):20–21, 1982.

18. Pironi L. and others. Relationship between intestinal per-

meability to 51-Cr EDTA and inflammatory activity in a-symptomatic patients with Crohn's disease. *Digestive Disease Science* 35(5):582–588, 1990.

19. Munkholm P. and others. Intestinal permeability in patients with Crohn's disease and ulcerative colitis and their first degree relatives. *Gut* 35(1):68–72, 1994.

20. Hollander D. and others. Increased intestinal permeability in patients with Crohn's disease and their relatives. A possible etiologic factor. *Annals of Internal Medicine* 105(6): 883–885, 1986.

21. Teahon K. and others. Intestinal permeability in patients with Crohn's disease and their first degree relatives. *Gut* 33(3):320–323, 1992.

22. Rooney P.J., Jenkins R.T., and Buchanan W.W. A short review of the relationship between intestinal permeability and inflammatory joint disease. *Clinical Experiments in Rheumatology* 8(1):75–83, 1990.

23. Jenkins R.T. and others. Increased intestinal permeability in patients with rheumatoid arthritis: a side-effect of oral nonsteroidal anti-inflammatory drug therapy? *British Journal of Rheumatology* 26(2):103–107, 1987.

24. Mielants H. Reflections on the link between intestinal permeability and inflammatory joint disease. Letter comment. *Clinical Experiments in Rheumatology* 8(5): 523–524, 1990.

25. Morris A.J. and others. Increased intestinal permeability in ankylosing spondylitis—primary lesion or drug effect? *Gut* 32(12):1470–1472, 1991.

26. Smith M.D., Gibson R.A., and Brooks P.M. Abnormal bowel permeability in ankylosing spondylitis and rheumatoid arthritis. *Journal of Rheumatology* 12(2): 299–305, 1985.

27. Skoldstam L. and Magnusson K.E. Fasting, intestinal permeability, and rheumatoid arthritis. *Rheumatic Disease Clinics of North America* 17(2):363–371, 1991.

28. Juhlin L. and Vahlquist C. The influence of treatment on fibrin microclot generation in psoriasis. *British Journal of Dermatology* 108(1):33–37, 1983.

29. Juhlin L. and Michaelson G. Fibrin microclot formation in patients with acne. *Acta Dermatologica Venereology* 63(6): 538–540, 1983.

30. Hamilton I. and others. Small intestinal permeability in dermatological disease. *Quarterly Journal of Medicine* 56(221): 559–567, 1985.

31. Belew P.W. and others. Endotoxemia in psoriasis. Letter. *Archives of Dermatology* 118(3):142–143, 1982.

32. Jackson P.G. and others. Intestinal permeability in patients with eczema and food allergy. *Lancet* 1(8233):1285–1286, 1981.

33. Scadding G. and others. Intestinal permeability to 51 Cr-labelled ethylenediaminetetraacetate in food-intolerant subjects. *Digestion* 42(2):104–109, 1989.

34. Jacobson P., Baker R., and Lessof M. Intestinal permeability in patients with eczema and food allergy. *Lancet* I: 1285–1286, 1981.

35. Falth-Magnusson K. and others. Gastrointestinal permeability in children with cow's milk allergy: effect of milk challenge and sodium cromoglycate as assessed with polyethyleneglycols (PEG 400 and PEG 1000). *Clinical Allergy* 16(6):543–551, 1986.

36. Falth-Magnusson K. and others. Gastroinestinal permeability in atopic and nonatopic mothers, assessed with different-sized polyethyleneglycols (PEG 400 and PEG 1000). *Clinical Allergy* 14(3):277–286, 1991.

37. Falth-Magnusson K. and others. Intestinal permeability in healthy and allergic children before and after sodium-cromoglycate treatment assessed with different-sized polyethyleneglycols (PEG 400 and PEG 1000). *Clinical Allergy* 14(3):277–286, 1984.

38. Jalonen T. Identical intestinal permeability changes in children with different clinical manifestations of cow's milk allergy. *Journal of Allergy and Clinical Immunology* 88(5): 737–742, 1991.

39. Barau E. and Dupont C. Modifications of intestinal permeability during food provocation procedures in pediatric

irritable bowel syndrome. *Journal of Pediatric Gastroenterology Nutrition* 11(1):72–77, 1990.

40. Paganelli R. and others. Intestinal permeability in irritable bowel syndrome. Effect of diet and sodium cromoglycate administration. *Annals of Allergy* 64(4): 377–380, 1990.

41. Marston W. Gut reactions. *Newsweek,* 17 November 1997, pp. 95, 99.

42. Lichtman S.N. and others. Hepatic injury associated with small bowel bacterial overgrowth in rats is prevented by metronidazole and tetracycline. *Gastroenterology* 100(2):513–519, 1991.

43. Braganza J.M. and others. Lipid peroxidation (free radical oxidation) products in bile from patients with pancreatic disease. *Lancet* 11:375–378, 1983.

44. Braganza J.M. and others. Pancreatic disease: a casualty of hepatic "detoxification"? *Lancet* ii:1000–1002, 1983.

45. Batash S. and others. Intestinal permeability in HIV infection: proper controls are necessary. Letter. *American Journal of Gastroenterology* 87(5):680, 1992.

46. Lim S.G. and others. Intestinal permeability and function in patients infected with human immunodeficiency virus. A comparison with coeliac disease. *Scandinavian Journal of Gastroenterology* 28(7):573–580, 1993.

47. Tepper R.E. and others. Intestinal permeability in patients infected with human immunodeficiency virus. *American Journal of Gastroenterology* 89:878–882, 1994.

48. Mack D.R. and others. Correlation of intestinal lactulose permeability with exocrine pancreatic dysfunction. *Journal of Pediatrics* 120:696–701, 1992.

49. Baker S. Introductory comments. In: *Dysbiosis: A Clinical Symposium.* Asheville NC: Great Smokies Diagnostic Laboratory, 1992, p. 1–4.

50. Galland L. Leaky gut syndromes: breaking the vicious cycle. In: *Solving the Digestive Puzzle.* San Francisco: Great Smokies Diagnostic Laboratory and HealthComm International, Inc., 1995, pp. 1–21.

CHAPTER 7

How The Yeast Syndrome Affects More Than Just the Digestive System

1. Trowbridge J.P. and Walker M. *The Yeast Syndrome.* New York: Bantam Books, 1986.

2. Burnhill M.S. Sorting out the major vaginal infections. *Contemporary OB/GYN,* April 1987, pp. 47–62.

3. Burnhill M.S. Taking a serious approach to vulvovaginitis. *Contemporary OB/GYN,* September 1986, pp. 69–79.

4. Burnhill M.S. Clinician's guide to counseling patients with chronic vaginitis. *Contemporary OB/GYN,* January 1990, pp. 37–44.

5. Rippon J.W. *Medical Mythology.* 2nd ed. Philadelphia: W.B. Saunders, 1982.

6. Crook W.G. *The Yeast Connection.* 3rd ed. Jackson MS: Professional Books, 1986, 47–48.

7. Trowbridge J.P. and Walker M. *Yeast-Related Illnesses.* Greenwich CT: Devin-Adair Publishers, 1987, p. 148.

CHAPTER 8

Intestinal Parasites and Chronic Illness

1. Thorne G.M. Diagnosis of infectious diarrheal diseases. *Infectious Diarrhea* 1:747–751, 1988.

2. Goncalves J.F., Tanabe M., Medeiros F.M., Goncalves F.J., Motta S.R.N., Tateno S., and Takeuchi T. Parasitological and serological studies on amoebiasis and other intestinal parasitic infections in the rural sector around Recife, Northeast Brazil. *Rev Inst Med Trop Sao Paulo* 32(6):428–435, 1990.

3. Dalton H.P. and Nottebart H.C. *Interpretive Medical Microbiology.* 1986, p. 501.

4. Kotulak R. Parasites more common than believed, study says. *Miami Herald* (Chicago Tribune Service), 27 June 1978.

5. Korelitz B.I. When should we look for amebae in patients with inflammatory bowel disease? *Journal of Clinical Gastroentrology* 11(4):373–375, 1989.

6. Radvin J.L. *Entamoeba histolytica*: From adherence to enteropathy. *Journal of Infectious Diseases* 159:420, 1989.

7. Balows A., Hausler W.J., Herrmann K.L., Isenberg H.D., and Shadomy H.J. *Manual of Clinical Microbiology*. 5th ed. American Association of Microbiology, 1991, pp. 702, 754–756.

8. Abu-Shakra M. Parasitic infectional autoimmunity. *Autoimmunity* 9(4):337–344, 1991.

9. Owen R.L. Parasitic disease. In: *Gastrointestinal Disease: Pathophysiology, Diagnosis, Management*. Philadelphia: Saunders, 1989, pp. 1402–1418.

10. Gittleman A.L. *Guess What Came to Dinner: Parasites and Your Health*. Garden City Park NY: Avery Publishing Group, 1993, pp. 9–10.

11. Smith P.D., Quinn T.C., Strober W., Janoff E.N., and Masur H. Gastrointestinal infections in AIDS. *Annals of Internal Medicine* 116:63–77, 1992.

12. Kotler D.P., Francisco A., Clayton F., Scholes J.Y.V.and Orenstein J.M. Small intestinal injury and parasitic diseases in AIDS. *Annals of Internal Medicine* 113:444–449, 1990.

13. Ash L.R. and Orihel T.C. *Atlas of Human Parasitology*. 2nd ed. Chicago: American Society of Clinical Pathologists, 1980.

14. Sun T. *Color Atlas and Textbook of Diagnostic Parasitology*. Igakau-Shoin, 1988.

15. Fleming C., Frye C., and Lee M.J. Morphology and frequency of occurrence of *Blastocystic hominis*. ASCP/ CAP spring meeting, 2–7 March 1991, Nashville TN.

16. Ziert, C.H. *Blastocystic hominis*—past and future. *Clinical Microbiology Reviews*, January 1991, pp. 61–79.

17. Babb R.R. and Wagener S. *Blastocystic hominis*—a potential intestinal pathogen. *Western Journal of Medicine* 151:518–519, 1989.

18. Yang J. and Scholten T.H. *Dientamoeba fragilis*: a review with notes on its epidemiology, pathogenicity, mode of transmission, and diagnosis. *American Journal of Tropical Medicine and Hygine* 26(1):16–22, 1977.

19. Kean B.H. and Malloch C.L. The neglected ameba: *Dientamoeba fragilis. American Journal of Digestive Diseases* II(9): 735–746, 1966.

20. Balows A., Hausler W.J., Herrmann K.L., Isenberg H.D., and Shadomy H.J. *Manual of Clinical Microbiology.* 5th ed. American Association of Microbiology, 1991, pp. 702, 754–756.

21. Galland L. and Lee M. High frequency of giardiasis in patients with chronic digestive complaints. *American Journal of Gastroenterology* 84:1181, 1989.

22. Gittleman A.L. *Guess What Came to Dinner: Parasites and Your Health.* Garden City Park NY: Avery Publishing Group, 1993, p. 45.

23. Markell E.K., Voge M., and John D.T. *Medical Parasitology.* 6th ed. Philadelphia: Saunders, 1986, p. 6.

CHAPTER 9

Achieving Digestive Health Through Proper Diet

1. Eaton S.B. and Konner M. Paleolithic nutrition. A consideration of its nature and current implications. *New England Journal of Medicine* 312:283–289, 1985.

2. Simopoulos A.P. Evolutionary aspects of diet: obesity and reference standards. In Van Itallie T. and Sim-opoulos A.P. (eds): *Obesity: New Directions in Assessment and Management.* Philadelphia: Charles Press, 1995.

3. Leaf A. and Weber P.C. Cardiovascular effects of omega-3 fatty acids. *New England Journal of Medicine* 318:549–547, 1988.

4. Igram C. and Gray J.K. *Eat Right or Die Young.* Cedar Rapids IA: Literary Visions, Inc., 1989, p. 10.

5. Cresta M., Ledermann S., Garnier A., Lombardo E., and Lacourly G. *Etude des consommations alimentaires des populations de onze regions de la communaute europeenne en vue de la determination des niveaux de contamination radioactive.* Report of the Centre d'Etude Nucleaire de Fotenay-aux-Roses, France. EURATOM, Commissariat a l'Energie Atomique, 1969.

6. Willett W.C. Diet and health: What should we eat? *Science* 264:532–537, 1994.

7. Klatz R. and Goldman R. *Stopping the Clock: Why Many of Us Will Live Past 100—and Enjoy Every Minute!* New Canaan CT: Keats Publishing, Inc., 1996, p. 225.

8. Mitscher L.A. and Dolby V. *The Green Tea Book.* Garden City Park NY: Avery Publishing Group, 1998, pp. 118–120.

9. Ratnayake W.M.N., Hollywood R., O'Grady E., and Pelletier F. Fatty acids in some common food items in Canada. *Journal of American College of Nutrition* 12:651–660, 1993.

10. Simopoulos A.P., Koletzko B., Anderson R.E., and others. Fatty acids and lipids from cell biology to human disease. *Journal of Lipid Research* 35:169–173, 1994.

11. Reaven P., Parthasarathy S., Grasse B.J., and others. Effects of oleate-enriched and linoleate-enriched diets on the susceptibility of low density lipoprotein to oxidative modification in hypercholesterolemic subjects. *Journal of Clinical Investigation* 91:668–676, 1993.

12. Leaf A. and Weber P.C. Cardiovascular effects of omega-3 fatty acids. *New England Journal of Medicine* 318:549–547, 1988.

CHAPTER 10

The Many Benefits of Yogurt

1. The yogurt chronicles. *International Fresh Daily,* www. yaourt. org/archives.html (17 October 1997).

2. Gilliland S.K.E. and Speck M.L. Antagonistic action of *Lactobacillus acidophilus* toward intestinal and foodborne pathogens in associative cultures. *Journal of Food Protection* 40: 820–823, 1977.

3. Fernandes C.F. and Shahani K.M. Modulation of antibiosis by lactobacilli and yogurt and its healthful and beneficial significance. In R.C. Chandan (ed.): *Yogurt: Nutritional and Health Properties.* McClean VA: National Yogurt Association, 1989, pp. 145–159.

4. *Journal of Dairy Science* 73:905, 1990.

5. Can yogurt lower blood cholesterol levels? *International Fresh Daily*, www.yaourt.org/hb_cholesterol.html (17 October 1997).

6. *Foods, Nutrition and Immunity* 1:77, 1992.

7. *American Journal of Clinical Nutrition* 39:756, 1984.

8. DeSimone C.B., Salvadori B., Jirillo E., Baldinelli L., Bitonti F., and Vesely R. Modulation of immune activities in humans and animals by dietary lactic acid bacteria. In R.C. Chandan (ed.): *Yogurt: Nutritional and Health Properties*. McClean VA: National Yogurt Association, 1989, pp. 201–213.

9. Halpern G.M., Vruwink K.G., Van de Water J., Keen C.L., and Gershwin M.E. Influence of long-term yoghurt consumption in young adults. *International Journal of Immunotherapy* 7(4):205–210, 1991.

10. Trapp and others. Cited in: Can yogurt boost your natural defenses? *International Fresh Daily* www.yaourt.org/hb_naturaldefense.html (17 October 1997).

11. Heeler L. Yogurt: Bring it back alive. *Hippocrates*, July/August 1991, pp. 21–24.

12. Hilton E. *Annals of Internal Medicine* 116:353, 1992.

13. Metchnikoff E. *The Prolongation of Life*. New York: G.P. Putnam and Sons, The Knickerbocker Press, 1908.

14. Walker M. *Secrets of Long Life*. Old Greenwich CT: Devin-Adair Publishing, 1983.

15. Walker M. Lively components of yogurt. *Townsend Letter for Doctors and Patients*, December 1993, pp. 1184–1187.

16. Sellars R.L. Health properties of yogurt. In R.C. Chandan (ed.): *Yogurt: Nutritional and Health Properties*. McLean VA: National Yogurt Association, 1989, pp. 115–144.

17. Chandan R.C. and Shahani K.M. Yogurt. In Y.H. Hui (ed.): *Dairy Science and Technology Handbook*. Vol. 2. McClean VA: National Yogurt Association, 1993, pp. 10–11.

18. Mitsuoka T. *Intestinal Bacteria and Health: An Introductory Narrative*. Tokyo: Harcourt Brace Jovanovich Japan, 1978, p. 91.

CHAPTER 11
Internal Cleansing for Intestinal Health

1. Digesting fiber. *Nutrition Action Healthletter* 21(7):6, 1994.

2. Liebman B. Fiber: Separating fact from fiction. *Nutrition Action Healthletter* 21(7):5, 1994.

3. Liebman B. Heart-saving fiber? *Nutrition Action Healthletter* 23(3):2, 1996.

4. Balch J.F. and Balch P.A. *Prescription for Nutritional Healing.* 2nd ed. Garden City Park NY: Avery Publishing Group, 1997, pp. 545–546.

5. Bounous G. Dietary whey protein inhibits the development of dimethylhydrazine induced malignancy. *Clinical Investigative Medicine* 12:213–217, 1988.

6. Hoffman R.L. *7 Weeks to a Settled Stomach.* New York: Pocket Books, 1991, pp. 226–227.

7. Darling P. and others. Protein quality and quantity in preterm infants receiving the same energy intake. *American Journal of Disabled Children* 139:186, 1985.

8. Raima N.C.R. and others. Milk protein quantity and quality in low birth weight infants: Metabolic responses and effects on growth. *Pediatrics* 57:659–674, 1976.

9. Leibovitz B. Whey protein, a unique source of protein. *Muscular Development Magazine*, 26, 1989.

10. Bounous G., Gervais F., Amer V., Batist G., and Gold P. The influence of dietary whey protein on tissue glutathione and the diseases of aging. *Clinical Investigative Medicine* 12, 1989.

11. Bounous G., Kongshavin P., and Gold P. The immunoenhancing property of dietary whey protein concentrate. *Clinical Investigative Medicine* 11:271–278, 1988.

12. Leibovitz B. Whey protein, a unique source of protein. *Muscular Development Magazine*, 1989.

13. Renner E. *Milk and Dairy Products in Human Nutrition.* Munich: Verlag W. Volkswirtschaftlicher, 1983, p. 104.

14. Bounous, G., Kongshavn P., and Gold P. The immunoen-

hancing property of dietary whey protein concentrate. *Clinical Investigative Medicine* 11:271–278, 1988.

15. Rosanne K., Fu Tsan M., and Fu Tsan F. Enhancement of intracellular glutathione promotes lymphocyte activation by mitogen. *Cellular Immunology* 97: 155–163, 1986.

16. Bounous G. and Gold P. The biological activity of undenatured dietary whey proteins: Role of glutathione. *Clinical Investigative Medicine* 14(4):296–309, 1991.

17. Webster D. *Colon Flora: The Missing Link in Immunity, Health & Longevity.* Cardiff CA: Hygeia Publishing, 1995.

18. Adetumbi M.A. and Lau B.H.S. Allium sativum (garlic) inhibits lipids synthesis by *Candida albicans. Antimicrobial Agents & Chemotherapy* 30:499–501, 1986.

19. Fructooligosaccharide information package. The AJS Company, Orange CA, May 1990.

CHAPTER 12

Banishing Indigestion for Good With Probiotics

1. Walker M. The value of acidophilus. *Explore!* 4(1):33, 1993.

2. Moss J. The many facets of intestinal microflora. *Moss Nutrition Newsletter,* No. 15, December 1995, p. 5.

3. Mitsuoka T. Bacteria in the intestines. *Medicina* 21(8):1374, 1984.

4. Mitsuoka T. Intestinal bacteria flora and its significance. *Clinics and Bacteria* 2(3):55, 1975.

5. Mitsuoka T. Effect of lactic acid bacteria and new application areas. *Journal of Japanese Food Industry* 31(4): 285, 1984.

6. Lee H., Friend B.A., and Shahani K.M. Factors affecting the protein quality of yogurt and acidophilus milk. *Journal of Dairy Science* 71:3203–3214, 1988.

7. Fernandes C.F., Shahani K.M., and Amer M.A. Therapeutic role of dietary lactobacilli and lactobacilli fermented dairy products. *FEMS Microbiology Review* 46:343–356, 1987.

8. Pollman D.S., Danielson D.M., Wren W.B., Peo E.R., and Shahani K.M. Influence of *Lactobacillus acidophilus* inoculum on guotobiotic and conventional pigs. *Journal of Ani-*

mal Science 51:629–637, 1980.

9. Yamamoto F. and others. Effect of lactic acid bacteria on intestinally decomposed substance-producing bacteria of human source. *Basics and Clinics* 20(14): 123, 1986.

10. Fernandes C.F. and Shahani K.M. Lactose intolerance and its modulation with lactobacilli and other microbial supplements. *Journal of Applied Nutrition* 41:50–64, 1989.

11. Filliland S.E. Health and nutritional benefits from lactic acid bacteria. *FEMS Microbiology Review* 87:175–188, 1990.

12. Honma A. On effects of lactic acid bacteria—No. 1: biological significance. *New Medicines and Clinics* 35(12):31, 1986.

13. Honma A. On effects of lactic acid bacteria—No. 2: clinical effects. *New Medicines and Clinics* 36(1):75, 1987.

14. Shahani K.M. and Ayebo A.D. Role of dietary lactobacilli in gastrointestinal microecology. *Journal of Clinical Nutrition* 33:2448–2457, 1980.

15. Rao D.R. and Shahani K.M. Vitamin content of cultured dairy products. *Cultured Dairy Products Journal* 22(1):6–10, 1987.

16. Kamen B. Consumer education series—cultured foods. *Health Foods Business*, October 1988, pp. 74–75.

17. Shahani K.M., Vakil J.R., and Kilara A. Natural antibiotic activity of *L. acidophilus* and *bulgaricus*. I. Cultural conditions for the production of antibiosis. *Cultured Dairy Products Journal* 11(4):14–17, 1976.

18. Shahani K.M., Vakil J.R., and Kilara A. Natural antibiotic activity of *L. acidophilus* and *bulgaricus*. II. Isolation of acidolophilia from *L. acidophilus*. *Cultured Dairy Products Journal* 12(2):8–11, 1977.

19. Shahani K.M., Vakil J.R., and Chandan R.C. Antibiotic acidophilus and the process for preparing the same. U.S. Patent 3,689,640. 5 September 1972.

20. Reddy G.V., Shahani K.M., Friend B.A., and Chandan R.C. Natural antibiotic acitivity of *L. acidophilus* and *bulgaricus*. III. Production and partial purification of bulgarican from *L. bulgaricus*. *Cultured Dairy Products Journal* 18(2):15–19, 1983.

21. Fernandes C.F., Shahani K.M., and Amer M.A. Control of diarrhea by lactobacilli. *Journal of Applied Nutrition* 40:32–43, 1988.

22. Fernandes C.F., Shahani K.M., and Amer, M.A. Effect of nutrient media and bile salts on growth and antimicrobial activity of *L. acidophilus*. *Journal of Dairy Science* 71: 3222–3228, 1988.

23. Chan R.C.Y., Reid G., Irvin R.T., Bruce A.W., and Costerton I.W. Competitive exclusion of uropathogens from human uroepithelial cells by Lactobacillus. *Infections and Immunity* 47:84–89, 1985.

24. Honma A. On effects of lactic acid bacteria—No. 1: biological significance. *New Medicines and Clinics* 35(12):31, 1986.

25. Honma A. Intestinal bacteria flora of infants and infection protection. *Pediatric Clinics* 27(11):20, 1974.

26. DeSimone C. and others. The adjuvant effect of yogurt on gamma interferon by Con-A stimulated human lymphocytes. *Nutritonal Reports International* 33: 419–433, 1986.

27. Perdigon G.and others. Effect of peritoneally administered lactobacilli on microphage. *Infection and Immunity* 53:404–410, 1986.

28. Shahani K.M., Fernandes C.F., and Amer M.A. Effect of yogurt on intestinal flora and immune responses. *Dairy Industry*, 1987, pp. 57–67.

29. Fernandes C.F. and Shahani K.M. Anticarcinogenic and immunological properties of dietary lactobacilli. *Journal of Food Protection* 53:704–710, 1990.

30. Fernandes C.F., Shahani, K.M., Staudinger W.L., and Amer M.A. Mode of tumor suppression by *Lactobacillus acidophilus*. *Journal of Nutrition and Medicine* 2: 25–34, 1991.

31. Bottazzi V., Friend B.A., and Shahani K.M. Properta antitumorali dei batteri lattici e degl. alimenti fermentati con batteri lactttici. *Il Latte* 10:873–879, 1985.

32. Honma A. On effects of lactic acid bacteria—No. 2: clinical effects. *New Medicines and Clinics* 36(1):75, 1987.

33. Honma A. On intestinal bacterial flora. *Pharmacology News* 8:21, 1987.

34. Kaup S.M., Shahani K.M., and Amer M.A. Bioavailability of calcium in yogurt. *Milchweissenschaft* 42: 513–516, 1987.

35. Danielson A.D., Peo E.R., Shahani K.M., Lewis A.J., Whalen P.J., and Amer M.A. Anticholesteremic property of *L. acidophilus* yogurt fed to mature boars. *Journal of Animal Science*, 64(4):966–974, 1989.

36. Yoneda H. Biological study on live bacteria products in the market. *Medicine and Pharmacology* 17(6):1529, 1987.

37. Honma A. On effects of lactic acid bacteria—No. 1: biological significance. *New Medicines and Clinics* 35(12):31, 1986.

38. Yamamoto F. and others. Effect of lactic acid bacteria on intestinally decomposed substance-producing bacteria of human source. *Basics and Clinics* 20(14): 123, 1986.

39. Ionescu G., Jeaht E.W., Linebeck R., and Shahani K.M. Orale lactobazillen bei atopischem ekzem. *Ortho Suppl* 2: 1–4, 1988.

40. Yutsis P. and Walker M. *The Downhill Syndrome.* Garden City Park NY: Avery Publishing Group, 1997, pp. 18–19.

41. Hilts P.J. President orders faster approval of cancer drugs. *The New York Times*, 30 March 1996, pp. 1,9.

42. Winter R. *Cancer-Causing Agents.* New York: Crown Publishing, 1991, p. 1.

43. Red hot meat. *Nutrition Action Healthletter* 22(2):13, 1995.

44. Winter R. *Cancer-Causing Agents.* New York: Crown Publishing, 1991, p. 150.

45. Winter R. *Cancer-Causing Agents.* New York: Crown Publishing, 1991, p. 151.

46. Mitsuoka T. *Intestinal Bacteria and Health.* Tokyo: Harcourt Brace Jovanovich Japan, Inc., 1978, pp. 161–163.

47. Mitsuoka T. *Intestinal Bacteria and Health.* Tokyo: Harcourt Brace Jovanovich Japan, Inc., 1978, pp. 148–150.

48. Goldin B.R., Swenson L., Dwyer J., Sexton M., and Gor-

bach S.L. Effect of diet and Lactobacillus acidophilus supplements on human fecal bacterial enzymes. *Journal of the National Cancer Institute* 64: 255–261, 1980.

49. Goldin B.R. and Gorbach S.L. Alterations of the intestinal microflora by diet, oral antibiotics, and Lactobacillus: Decreased production of free amines from aromatic nitro compounds, azo dyes, and glucur onides. *Journal of the National Cancer Institute* 73(3): 689–695, 1984.

50. *Technical Bulletin*. Klaire Laboratories, Inc., June 1988, p. 2.

51. Branscum V. Intestinal flora and human health. *Explore!* 7(1):48, 1996.

Conclusion

1. Moss J. The many faces of intestinal microflora (Part IV). *Moss Nutrition Newsletter,* no. 115, December 1995.

Index